MW00388379

Overcoming Positional Vertigo

Carol A. Foster, MD

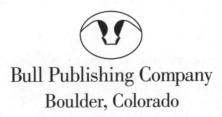

Bull Publishing Company
Boulder, Colorado

Copyright © 2019 by Carol A. Foster

All rights reserved. No part of this publication may be reproduced, distributed, or transmitted in any form or by any means, including photocopying, recording, or other electronic or mechanical methods, without the prior written permission of the publisher, except in the case of brief quotations embodied in critical reviews and certain other noncommercial uses permitted by copyright law.

Bull Publishing Company
P.O. Box 1377
Boulder, CO USA 80306
www.bullpub.com

Library of Congress Cataloging-in-Publication Data

Names: Foster, Carol A., author.
Title: Overcoming positional vertigo / Carol A Foster, MD.
Description: Boulder, CO : Bull Publishing Company, [2019] |
    Includes bibliographical references and index.
Identifiers: LCCN 2018049530 | ISBN 9781945188176 (paperback)
Subjects: LCSH: Vertigo--Treatment. | Vertigo—Diagnosis. | BISAC:
HEALTH & FITNESS / Diseases / General. | SELF-HELP / General.
Classification: LCC RB150.V4 F67 2019 | DDC 616.8/41—dc23
LC record available at https://lccn.loc.gov/2018049530

Printed in the U.S.A.

23 22 21 20 19 18   10 9 8 7 6 5 4 3 2 1

Interior design and production by Dovetail Publishing Services
Cover design and production by Shannon Bodie, Bookwise Design

To all those who suffer from vertigo and to my family for their loving support of my efforts to alleviate dizziness.

Disclaimer

This book does not replace professional medical diagnosis or treatment. I encourage you to seek the advice of your health care provider with any questions you have regarding your health. Do not delay seeing a medical provider when you become ill and be sure to follow any treatment instructions you are given.

Contents

Preface

Vertigo is a worthy foe, and my aim is to end it.

Strangely, a lot of people think it's fun to spin and happily seek out thrilling rides that make them dizzy for a few moments. It's a completely different matter when the spinning comes of its own volition, without warning. It attacks vision, making the world a whirling blur. It attacks balance, making some victims crawl instead of walk. It magnifies the indignity by adding in nausea and vomiting. It makes people lose faith in themselves, no longer able to trust that their eyes will always see clearly or that their limbs will always support them. They begin to fear going out in public, driving cars, exercising, or even simply lying down in bed. It isolates people because it is something only the sufferer can feel, with few signs to alert others to the magnitude of the horror they endure. In my medical practice, I am privileged to see only dizziness patients. My dedicated partners at the University of Colorado Denver care for the rest of the diseases of the ears and brain so I can devote all my time to these uniquely suffering people.

Most people can overcome their dizziness, so as I listen to their stories I also watch intently for clues that they have a curable disease. About a third of my patients start their descriptions by relating that dizziness came on when they were in bed. This is the best story to hear, because it often means they have the most easily treated form of vertigo. I devote an entire clinic each week to this one disease:

positional vertigo. It's long been my most popular clinic with medical residents and fellows learning how to treat dizziness because the outcome is so positive. Most people with positional vertigo leave the clinic free of symptoms, no matter how severe it was when they arrived. I love to see tears replaced by smiles and hugs.

The problem is that vertigo is common and there are too few professionals who can treat it. People write me from all over the world asking if I know someone near them who can help. Medical care is often too expensive or access to trained specialists is too restricted for them to find a solution to their problem. The wonderful news is that for the most common vertigo disorder—a form of vertigo brought on by certain movements—it is possible to treat the problem at home, for free, and in just minutes, without having to find a trained specialist or pay for a clinic visit. This is why I wrote this book.

Acknowledgments

This book did not spring forth unbidden but arose from the generous mentoring, encouragement, and assistance of many dedicated people.

I want to start with the college professor who taught me the beauty of writing: Dr. Noel Riley Fitch. You were a dynamic and inspiring person to all of us who were privileged to learn from you. Thank you for sharing your talents, inspiration, and friendship over these many years.

Dr. Jeffrey P. Harris, otologist extraordinaire, you taught me that an ear could be beautiful. When I was suffering, you relieved me.

Dr. Robert W. Baloh, the ideal archetype of a gentleman of learning, it fell to you to teach me about the world of dizziness diseases. There could be no more perfect mentor.

I am indebted to the audiologists whose professionalism and caring natures help calm suffering patients. Kathleen Zaccaro, you know how much I have treasured your knowledge and skill. Darcy, Laura, Barbie, Donna, and Jennifer, thanks to all of you for working every day to make the sick feel better.

My publisher, Jim Bull of Bull Publishing, our first meeting felt like it was pre-destined. I deeply appreciate the opportunity you provided me to help dizzy people through this book. I also wish to thank Jon Peck for producing this work while dealing gracefully with a forest of little alterations.

Books are made by editors, and I am privileged to have great ones: Erin Mulligan and Julianna Scott Fein. You were magically able to give clarity to my written thoughts without losing key content. Thank you for the fortitude to re-read the manuscript so many times and with such care.

To our artist Joanne Brummett, the artwork is critical to make a complex subject understandable. You have my admiration for your ability to turn my sketches and scribbles into beautiful works of art.

Finally, I wish to thank my family. My husband Dr. Robert Breeze has always been the sounding board for my ideas and the first to edit my writings. Our daughters have been enthusiastic in their support and encouragement even though they know I am only pretending to be listening to them sometimes. I promise to do better.

1

An Introduction to Benign Paroxysmal Positional Vertigo (BPPV)

❝ There was no reason for trouble to start. I was sitting in a restaurant in Maui, chased indoors by heavy rains, looking forward to lunch and a piña colada. No sooner had the food arrived, without any warning, I suddenly felt a horrible twisting inside my head. I felt like I was being pulled out of my chair to the side and flipped over all at the same time. I grabbed the chair seat with both hands and managed to keep from falling off of the chair onto the restaurant floor. I looked around the restaurant and no one else seemed to be acting unusual. Nothing was moving except inside my head. The spinning stopped about 15 minutes later, returned briefly a few days later, and then disappeared for four months. But then it started to come back often and lasted 30 minutes, an hour, several hours at a time. Gradually, it was happening almost every day. During the worse spells, I could see the room shifting about me, and I noticed odd sounds and feelings in one ear, including roaring noises, clanking, and a sensation of stuffiness.

After a year of this torture, something new happened. One morning, when I rolled over in bed toward the bad ear, it felt like the room began to spin intensely. It was more violent than any of the prior spells but stopped after about 30 seconds. Trying to get out of bed set it off again, however, so I was only able to get out of bed when I moved very slowly. That morning, I went to see an ENT I had worked with previously, and he diagnosed Benign Paroxysmal Positional Vertigo (BPPV), but he also expressed concern that I had more going on in the bad ear than just BPPV. After experiencing months of BPPV spells and the daily vertigo, I had begun to lose hearing in the bad ear and was ultimately diagnosed with Meniere's disease. **"**

My Vertigo Journey and the Half Somersault

At that moment, when I experienced vertigo on Maui, my entire life shifted and it would never be the same again. It was especially cruel because I was a physician, trained in otolaryngology, the field that deals with vertigo, so I had treated many people with these vertigo disorders and knew from my clinical experience just how horrible these disorders could be. There weren't many treatments that seemed to help, and I had witnessed the sufferers coming in again and again seeking help in their misery. Now I was one of them.

Over the next few years, I suffered from severe vertigo (a disease called Meniere's disease) until I was rescued by my residency mentor, Dr. Jeff Harris, who finally cut the nerve to my bad ear so it could no longer make me spin. What I had learned about vertigo as a physician didn't come close to matching what I learned from personally experiencing it. It was much, much worse than I ever imagined before it happened to me, and it became my life's mission to help as many other people with vertigo as possible. To that end, I did a fellowship in neuro-otology at UCLA with Dr. Robert Baloh and Dr. Vicente Honrubia, who had written a key textbook on vertigo disorders and taught me all the latest knowledge of vestibular diseases.

I moved to the University of Colorado in 1994 and began treating dizziness and imbalance. One of the most common dizziness problems was positional vertigo (dizziness in certain head positions), and I tested every patient for this. At the time, very few people in Colorado knew that it was most often a small mechanical problem involving crystals in the ears and could usually be treated with a simple maneuver. Over the years, I first saw hundreds, and eventually thousands, of sufferers and conducted the treatment maneuver and its variations many thousands of times. The ability to relieve an awful disease using your bare hands is so very unusual in medicine, and I enjoyed doing it as much as my patients loved being helped. There was one problem with this kind of positional vertigo, though: Even though it can often be cured by a simple maneuver, it can also easily happen again. Many patients would ultimately need another treatment, some would need to be treated over and over. I tried giving patients various maneuvers as home exercises to cure recurrences, but patients still returned because the home maneuvers did not help them enough. After more than a decade of seeking, I hadn't found the perfect home treatment. That changed in 2006, when I discovered the Half Somersault maneuver.

The discovery was serendipitous. I was getting up one morning to go to work and treat people in my vertigo clinic. When I rolled over in bed, I suddenly developed positional vertigo in my "good" ear. This had never happened to me before, and I knew it meant that I had dislocated some crystals into the wrong part of my ear. I tried to do the usual office maneuvers and ended up getting the crystals into other places in my ear that caused even more severe vertigo. I crawled back into bed with a bucket in case I got sick and tried to figure out an alternative. Using my fingers as rings I constructed a little model of the inner ear and moved it around to see if there was a way to remove the crystals more easily. After a few minutes I realized that a modified somersault position should work. I got down on the floor and did the Half Somersault maneuver for the first time. I arose completely free of vertigo.

Naturally, I added this exercise to the others I was already "prescribing" as home treatments. Patients that took the other exercises home often came back with recurrences, but those using the Half Somersault did not. This led me to assemble a team to perform a study of the new exercise. Our evidence-based research paper showing the effectiveness of the Half Somersault was published in 2012,[1] and since then millions of people have downloaded videos and handouts of the exercise for home use.

What Is Benign Paroxysmal Positional Vertigo (BPPV)?

The most common vertigo disorder is Benign Paroxysmal Positional Vertigo, which we commonly refer to as BPPV. Although there are many ailments that cause vertigo, it is only this particular disorder—BPPV—that can be relieved using simple maneuvers. BPPV does not require surgery, medications, or prolonged physical therapy to treat; in most people, the vertigo caused by BPPV can be stopped in a matter of minutes. In BPPV, heavy crystals that are normally used by the ear to detect the pull of gravity accidentally fall into one of the spinning sensors of the inner ear. By placing the head in just the right position, the crystals can be shaken back out, restoring normal function and ending the symptoms of vertigo almost instantly.

The typical symptoms of BPPV are easy to recognize: The world spins briefly when you make certain rapid head movements. The vertigo can be severe enough to cause nausea and vomiting. Most BPPV spells occur around bedtime or when you are getting out of bed in the morning and improve once you are upright. However, some people continue to feel mildly off balance during the day. Hearing is not affected by this disorder. While most forms of BPPV cause this relatively mild pattern of vertigo, there are some forms of BPPV that cause more severe and prolonged vertigo (I cover these forms later in this book).

BPPV can occur in children, but the number of people with symptoms begins to rise steadily with age starting around age 30, and by age 60 about 10% of people experience this vertigo. Overall, more than two people out of every hundred will experience BPPV during their lifetimes; of more than 7 billion people on earth, this means over 150 million already have or will one day experience this disease. Women are twice as likely to get BPPV as men.

How Do I Know if I Have BPPV?

The key symptoms of BPPV are very short spells of vertigo—less than a minute long—that are brought on by head movement. Spells are more likely to happen around bedtime than during the day, and are brought on by rolling over in bed, lying down in bed, or arising quickly from a lying down position. Tipping the head up, as you might do when reaching up to a top shelf or screwing in an overhead bulb, can set it off. I created this book to be a resource and a tool for people to figure out if they have BPPV and potentially treat

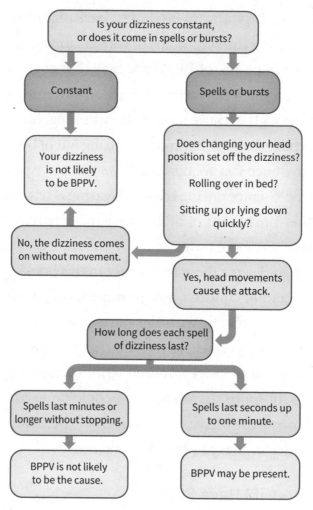

Figure 1.1 Symptoms chart.

themselves at home. The flow chart in Figure 1.1 will help you decide if your symptoms of dizziness are due to BPPV.

Treatment for BPPV and How to Use This Book

BPPV is a mechanical disorder of the ear, and therefore it is treated mechanically with maneuvers that involve certain head positions. Fortunately, there is no pain during treatment, but it does stir up the dizziness briefly. Medications can be used to reduce this dizziness while the maneuvers are done, but there are no medications that "cure" BPPV.

In the century since it was first identified, physicians learned early on that moving the head sometimes resolved the dizziness stemming from BPPV. However, it was only a few decades ago that the first "instant" treatments were created—the Epley and (later) the Semont maneuvers. These maneuvers (named after the physicians that popularized them) are usually performed by trained providers such as a physician, audiologist, or physical therapist. The Epley maneuver and the Semont maneuver are covered in detail in Chapter 10, "Maneuvers Performed by a Provider." As this book is a tool for people to potentially treat their BPPV at home, most readers who pick up this book will no doubt be looking for an easy home remedy for their symptoms. To that end, Chapter 7, "The Half Somersault Maneuver," and Chapter 8, "Variations on the Half Somersault Maneuver," cover the Half Somersault maneuver, which I developed in my own medical practice, and its variations. These exercises are intended for home treatment. Over the years, researchers have continued to learn about less common varieties of BPPV and have devised new maneuvers for these specific variations. These treatments, which are usually performed by trained therapists, are found in Chapter 9, "Unusual Forms of BPPV."

Understanding the process that results in vertigo spells depends on knowing the anatomy and physiology of the vestibular system—the sensors, brain pathways, and reflexes that control balance and sense motion. The next chapter introduces the key anatomy and also introduces the discoveries that gradually allowed physicians to find out what caused BPPV and to find ways to treat it.

2

The History of BPPV

"In the early hours of the morning, you snuggle half-asleep into the blankets and begin to roll over, as you have safely done countless times before, but this time something suddenly goes · horribly wrong. You feel an intense twisting and pulling as if your head is flipping in a circle. The feeling intensifies in the next few seconds into a violent, head-over-heels spinning. You feel like you are about to fly off the bed in a spiral, and you struggle to grab a handful of sheets to ground yourself. Your heart is pounding. You open your eyes and the world appears to be spinning so fast it's just a blur. You're vaguely aware that you have just rolled over and you turn your head back to try to undo whatever it was that set off this nightmare. Almost magically, the spinning stops, as if a switch has been shut off.

You lie there perfectly still, afraid to move for fear you will set it all off again. The panic that arrived with the spinning makes you feel shaky, and it's hard to calm down because you don't know what just happened. Are you having a stroke or heart attack? Are you going to pass out? Or worse—is this what death feels like? It doesn't take long to realize, though, that nothing else is happening and that you are not going to faint. You're feeling queasy and decide to get up to visit the bathroom, but

9

as soon as you try to get out of bed, you endure another identical spell that almost flings you back onto the bed. It quickly becomes clear that moving your head triggers the spells. You carefully prop yourself up on a pillow and call for help. **"**

Defining Vertigo and Benign Paroxysmal Positional Vertigo (BPPV)

Although the first attack might convince you that your demise is imminent, you have likely just experienced a type of *positional dizziness,* a simple mechanical disorder that is one of the most common and least serious forms of vertigo. A number of forms of *vertigo,* the sensation of whirling and loss of balance, exist (Table 2.1). Vertigo creates an illusion of a spinning motion inside the head when there is no actual head movement going on. The spinning that some little kids like to set off by spinning on their feet and suddenly stopping is a form of vertigo. Two or three people out of a hundred experience

Table 2.1 BPPV can be distinguished from other inner ear diseases by its symptoms.

Symptom	BPPV	Other vertigo diseases
Length of vertigo spell	Room spins for seconds, repeats	Constant spinning for more than 5 minutes
Trigger for vertigo spell	Head movement, usually vertical	Happens even if head is still
Time of day of vertigo spell	Around bedtime	Daytime when up and about
Other symptoms	None	Hearing loss, tinnitus, headache

at least one attack of positional dizziness during their lifetime, and episodes become more common with aging, eventually affecting up to 10% of the elderly.[1] This type of positional dizziness, and the unusually fast sensation of spinning it produces, isn't fatal and doesn't cause any permanent damage to the ear or brain, but it feels particularly frightening because it is one of the most intense forms of vertigo you can experience.

The disorder that results in the most common form of positional dizziness was originally named *benign paroxysmal positional vertigo*, but this has fortunately been abbreviated to BPPV. Let's look carefully at the name of this disorder and break it down to learn more about BPPV. While other types of vertigo can be damaging to the balance system, BPPV is *benign* because this type of vertigo is not associated with hearing loss or damage to the balance system (and is not at all fatal). BPPV is *paroxysmal*, meaning that it comes in sudden brief spells that last just a few seconds. Most other forms of vertigo last longer, from minutes to days at a time. BPPV is *positional*, brought on by changes in the position of the head in space, in contrast to other forms of vertigo or dizziness that can come on without any movement of the head at all (see Figure 1.1 on page 6). Finally, BPPV is most assuredly a form of *vertigo* because it results in an intense feeling of rotation inside the head even when the head is being held perfectly still.

BPPV in Human History

Humans have been experiencing BPPV for millennia. BPPV occurs in other animals, too, and has been clearly shown experimentally to affect cats,[2] but humans are more susceptible and far more likely to be diagnosed than other animals. BPPV is caused by a malfunction

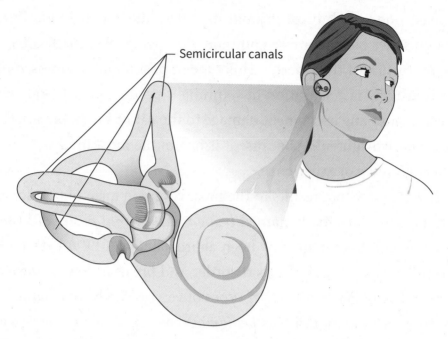

Semicircular canals

Figure 2.1   The semicircular canals of the inner ear are fluid-filled rings. There are three canals in each inner ear that create a three-dimensional arrangement to sense turning. Movement of the fluid is detected by the sensor.

in one of the spinning sensors in the inner ear. The sensor involved is one of the three *semicircular canals* in each of our ears (Figure 2.1), a tiny curved tube filled with fluid that first arose in early chordates (including the vertebrates, which are animals with backbones) over 300 million years ago. This sensor arose as a way to sense head movement.[3] Ideally, the sensor turns on only when the head is rotated; if it turns on when no rotation is taking place, this causes vertigo.

Even the words used to describe the experience of BPPV are ancient. The word *vertigo* derives from the Latin word *vertere,* meaning "to turn," and has been in use for at least 2,000 years. The Latin root is in turn derived from an even older Indo-European stem word *wert-, wer-,* or *wel-* meaning "to turn or rotate." Later, the "w" was changed to a "v" in some words. This stem gave rise to other English words with circular or spinning connotations, such as *wreath, vortex,* and *whirlpool.*[4]

The term *vertigo* is used in Latin sources to describe the sensation of spinning brought on by excessive drinking, a feeling that is still all too well-known today. The word *vertigo* languished during the Dark Ages but was rediscovered with a resurgence of interest in classical writings during the Renaissance and entered the English language in the Middle Ages. In the meantime, English speakers had to make do with the word *dizzy,* which referred more to a feeling of being stunned or dazed. Now both words—vertigo and dizziness—are used interchangeably. Until the nineteenth and twentieth centuries, no one made an effort to distinguish among the different dizziness disorders and they were generally all lumped together and referred to as *vertigo.*

"Discovering" BPPV

In fact, while people were no doubt experiencing BPPV symptoms for thousands of years, no one wrote down a clear description of the disorder until 1921.[5] The identification of BPPV is attributed to Dr. Robert Bárány (1876–1936), a Viennese physician who specialized in *vestibular disorders,* diseases of the ear and brain that can cause dizziness (Figure 2.2 on the next page). By the time he described BPPV, Bárány had already won the Nobel Prize for his explanation of the *caloric reaction,* a test that is still used to evaluate inner ear function.[6] It was once quite common for diseases to be named after the person who first described them, called an *eponym,* and in the past, there was considerable competition to achieve this recognition. Most discoveries depend upon clues that have been reported in earlier papers,

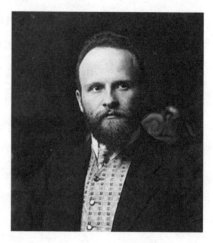

Figure 2.2   Dr. Robert Bárány is the only vestibular researcher to have won a Nobel Prize.

and an eponym tends to effectively erase the work of many researchers who supplied pieces of the puzzle leading to the final recognition of a disease. It is difficult to remember what the disease means if the name of it does not contain a clue. It can also be an annoyance for people with the same last name who don't want to appear to be named after a disease (for example, what if your last name actually was Alzheimer?). For these reasons, the trend over time has been to name diseases using descriptive terms and to avoid eponyms. BPPV was ahead of its time because it was given a descriptive name and was not named after Bárány. However, interestingly enough, most of the treatments for BPPV are now known by their eponyms. One of the reasons I named the Half Somersault maneuver so descriptively was that the name conveys key information about how the exercise is done.

BPPV is a very simple mechanical disorder in which crystals in the ear that are used to sense gravity fall into a spinning sensor. It seems like the cause of BPPV could have been figured out almost as soon as it was recognized. However, the course of scientific discovery is seldom smooth. It is very unusual for a new disorder to be depicted fully in the first paper written about it. An ideal scientific paper about a disease describes the symptoms and provides anatomical descriptions that explain the symptoms completely. Most of the time, however, only a few key aspects of the disease are initially described, and later papers by other authors fill in the remaining details. This process can take many years of study and a large number of researchers may be involved. In the case of BPPV, the process took nearly 60 years and researchers from all over the world contributed small bits of knowledge. There were a number of mistakes in the early papers that were discovered and overturned by later researchers. This delayed a full understanding of the disease. In this way, BPPV is an excellent example of the slow march of science.

All of the scientists who contributed to our understanding of BPPV were highly trained and intelligent, and many of them made discoveries about other conditions. So it may seem surprising that it took so long to figure out what was going on in this fairly simple disorder. However, each link in the chain of discovery depended on clues that only became available as time passed. Until the key clues were published or discussed, even keen scientists could not leap ahead to the final answer. This disease was identified by men and women working at universities around the world, not by a flash of insight by just one person. In the material that follows, we discuss the significant discoveries and the most obvious false leads.

By Bárány's time (the beginning of the 1900s), researchers had been doing experiments on the inner ears of animals for half a century. The opening in the skull behind the ear is so complex and intricate that anatomists originally named it the *labyrinth* (Figure

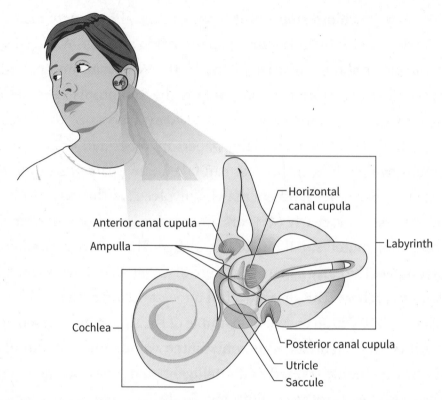

Horizontal
canal cupula

Anterior canal cupula

Ampulla

Labyrinth

Cochlea

Posterior canal cupula

Utricle

Saccule

Figure 2.3 Diagram of the membranous labyrinth. The labyrinth senses motion and the cochlea detects sound.

2.3). As time passed, scientists learned that the inner ears each have five sensors: two gravity sensors, called the *utricle* and *saccule*, and three spinning sensors, the semicircular canals. The gravity sensors work thanks to some relatively heavy particles that are clumped on the sensors that function by shifting or pressing down. This allows animals (like humans) to tell which way is down. The three canals are called the anterior, the horizontal, and the posterior semicircular canals. Each semicircular canal has a bulge, called the *ampulla*, at one end. Within each ampulla, there is a dividing flange (a fan-shaped moving flap) called the *cupula*. The movement of the cupula senses spinning. Whenever an animal's head is rotated, fluid in the canal moves and causes the cupula to move in response.

A number of researchers working with the ear had noticed that *nystagmus*, a jerking, spinning movement of the eyes, could be induced by rotating the heads of healthy people. Nystagmus also occurs without any associated head movement in people with inner ear diseases. Nystagmus is often observed in people suffering from vertigo. By the time BPPV was first reported, the directions of the eye movement in people suffering from nystagmus had been described and related to different diseases. The movement of the eyes (horizontal, vertical, torsional, or in combined directions) varied depending upon whether the head was moved slowly or quickly, the position of the head in space, and the relationship of the head movement to neck rotation. Bárány had a particular interest in these areas of study, so when his assistant, Dr. John Karlefors, came to see him with a patient with a new vertigo problem, he immediately tested her for these different forms of nystagmus.

"My assistant, Dr. Karlefors, first noticed that the attacks only occurred when she lay on her right side," he reported. "When she did this, there appeared a strong rotary nystagmus to the right. The attack lasted 30 seconds and was accompanied by violent vertigo and nausea."[7] Bárány noted that the attacks were brought on when she lay down, that they were brief, and that her pupils made repeated fast arcing and spinning movements during nystagmus.

He also noted that her nystagmus *fatigued* (weakened and wore off) if her head were repeatedly turned to the right while lying down, and after fatiguing, the response took some time before becoming activated again. Another key observation Bárány made was that the patient's hearing and central balance functions were normal. Bárány initially thought he was observing a disorder of the semicircular

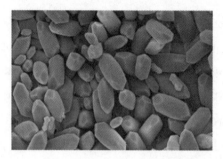

Figure 2.4   Otoconia. Gravity is sensed by the movement of these tiny chalk-powder crystalline particles that shift on top of a sensor in the ear.

canals. That was a correct assumption, but in the same paper Bárány changed his mind and blamed the disease on *otoliths*, which are, in humans, usually called *otoconia* (Figure 2.4). Otoconia are the heavy particles mentioned earlier that help the utricle and saccule sense gravity and tilt. Several decades later, both of Bárány's assumptions were found to be correct—the disorder does stem from a problem with the canals and the otoconia—but not in the way Bárány originally surmised. Because otoconia reside on two gravity sensors—most notably the utricle—in the inner ear, Bárány and others thought that a gravity sensor itself caused the symptoms of BPPV. This was not correct. While otoconia *are* involved, malfunction of the utricle is not the cause of vertigo in BPPV.

Dr. Carl-Olof Siggesson Nylén had worked with Bárány and several years later wrote a paper in which he described nystagmus that was set off when a patient's head was dangled off the end of a table, a head-hanging position that would later be important in diagnosing BPPV. However, Nylén did not describe the disorder in detail or differentiate it from other forms of vertigo, and his description of the head-hanging position was not detailed enough to allow others to easily identify Bárány's positional vertigo disorder.[8] However, some people still call the maneuver used to diagnose BPPV the Nylen–Barany maneuver to honor his contribution.

Shortly after BPPV was described, physicians observed that the problem tended to gradually go away on its own over the course of a few weeks in most people. But they could not figure out why it lasted much longer in some people or why it kept returning in new attacks. These attacks could be very disabling, so a method to treat it was in demand. The first treatment involved having patients simply avoid making the movements that set it off and be careful when the vertigo inevitably struck. People suffering from BPPV were told to lie down very slowly and to sit on the edge of the bed after arising to prevent falls if the vertigo occurred. Some sufferers learned to sleep sitting propped up on pillows, or with the head of the bed elevated, since this seemed to reduce the vertigo.

The Cawthorne–Cooksey Exercises

Sir Terence Cawthorne, an otologist at King's College Hospital and a sought-after consultant at many London hospitals from the 1920s through the 1960s, along with a specialist in rehabilitation medicine, Dr. F. S. Cooksey, developed an early treatment method for the symptoms of BPPV.[9] Cawthorne was eventually elected to the Presidency of the Royal Society of Medicine and was knighted for his efforts on behalf of patients. During World War II, numerous men with head injuries, many of whom had BPPV, experienced vertigo. To treat these soldiers, Cawthorne and Cooksey worked together to develop a plan for all kinds of vertigo that involved head and eye movements for the patients to perform when lying in bed, then while they were seated, and finally while standing and moving. Their method was published in 1946 and is still used to date. Some of the Cooksey and

Cawthorne exercises have been incorporated into more detailed modern programs of vestibular rehabilitation.

Many of the Cawthorne and Cooksey exercises were designed for those with permanent vestibular injuries, such as nerve damage after skull fracture. When Cooksey and Cawthorne came up with their exercises, no one was aware of the mechanical nature of the cause of BPPV, and most did not differentiate BPPV from other vertigo disorders. The Cawthorne–Cooksey exercises included rolling back and forth in bed, tipping the head up and down, and bending over from the seated position to retrieve an object on the floor. These movements were sufficient to move particles in the semicircular canals and to occasionally displace them back out. So even though Cooksey and Cawthorne did not know why the exercises worked, they still came up with a remedy that helped many people. Because BPPV tends to resolve on its own, especially in people who actively move the head, the Cawthorne–Cooksey exercises proved to be effective in treating BPPV.

The Dix–Hallpike Maneuver

In 1952, Dr. Margaret R. Dix and Dr. Charles S. Hallpike, who worked at the National Hospital in otology and were colleagues of Dr. Cawthorne in London, reviewed several papers on BPPV including those of Bárány and Nylen. The same year, Dix and Hallpike published the first thorough report in English about several vertigo disorders including positional vertigo. They named this "positional vertigo of the benign paroxysmal type," to differentiate it from other forms of positional vertigo that arise from more damaging causes and that cause continuous dizziness rather than short, violent bursts of vertigo.[10,11] This name was later shortened to benign paroxysmal positional vertigo and ultimately to the initials BPPV.

The most important feature of the 1952 Dix and Hallpike paper was a detailed description of how to diagnose the disease using a maneuver similar to that used by Bárány and Nylen. "The patient is laid supine upon a couch with his head just over its end. The head is then lowered some 30 degrees below the level of the couch and turned some 30 degrees to 45 degrees to one side. In taking up this position, the patient is first seated upon the couch with the head turned to one side and the gaze fixed upon the examiner's forehead. The examiner then grasps the patient's head firmly between his hands and briskly pushes the patient back into the critical position."[12] When this movement is done, BPPV is typically triggered. Because the patient is lying face up, the position makes it easy for the examiner to observe any nystagmus. This maneuver has become the definitive test for this condition (Figure 2.5). Over time, Dix and Hallpike were honored with an eponym for this maneuver, now most frequently called the *Dix–Hallpike maneuver* (or occasionally, the *Nylen–Barany maneuver*) or the shorter *Hallpike maneuver*. To this day the Dix–Hallpike maneuver is used to test for BPPV.

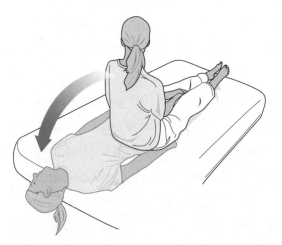

Figure 2.5 Dix–Hallpike maneuver. The seated patient is made to lie down with the head turned toward the shoulder at a 45-degree angle. The head is dropped off the end of the bed so that it is hanging downward. If BPPV is present, nystagmus is observable a few seconds after this position is achieved.

In their paper, Dix and Hallpike combined their review with additional clinical observations they had made of patients with vertigo. Like Bárány, they confirmed that the nystagmus was paroxysmal—coming in a violent burst—and that the course of the disorder was benign. There was no damage to hearing or any evidence of brain disease. They described in more detail the head movements that trigger spells. Lying down in bed, tipping the head upward, and rolling over in bed were cited as common triggers. Dix and Hallpike agreed with previous observers that the response tended to fatigue (weaken or disappear) with repetition.

Dix and Hallpike also noticed something that Bárány and Nylen had not mentioned. They noticed a lag of several seconds after the maneuver is done before the nystagmus appears, a characteristic called *latency*. They also added some key details to the description of the nystagmus. In particular, they noticed that when the patient was lying down with the head hanging to one side, the eyes appeared to be beating toward the floor. In the same paper they described how they proved with further experiments that the affected ear was the one that was downward in this triggering head position. This finding has been confirmed to be the case in the most common type of BPPV by all subsequent researchers. There are other types of BPPV that can be triggered when the affected ear is up, but this was not understood for many decades.

Dix and Hallpike published a review of 100 patients and an autopsy specimen of one person with BPPV. However, they still did not happen upon the correct explanation for the attacks. Bárány had thought that the vertigo spells were caused by the gravity sensors, and Dix and Hallpike agreed, even though this would turn out to be incorrect. Dix and Hallpike attributed the attacks to problems with the utricle or the saccule, the two gravity sensors in the inner ear, and failed to identify a key finding that would lead to a treatment 40 years later: that damage to the utricle can cause the release of otoconia, and it is the otoconia that cause the dizziness; the damage to the gravity sensor itself does not cause a spinning feeling.

Locating the Problem

The next advance occurred only four years later. In 1956, Dr. Garth Hemenway, an otology resident who would later become chief at the University of Colorado Department of Otolaryngology, and his mentor Dr. John R. Lindsay, a Canadian otologist at the University of Chicago,[13] published a paper describing severe degeneration of the utricle in several patients who developed repeated recurrences of BPPV following a sudden loss of function in other parts of the ear.[14] In these patients, although the utricle was no longer functioning and therefore could not be the source of the ongoing spells of vertigo, the posterior semicircular canal and saccule were still intact and still capable of being the source of vertigo. This finding meant that Bárány, Dix, and Hallpike could not be correct: The utricle was not the source of the vertigo spells. The spells had to be coming from the posterior semicircular canal or from the saccule (Figure 2.6 on the next page).

A review of the work by Hemenway and Lindsay led to the next major advance. It was a paper published in 1962, written by one of the more prominent otologists in the world, Harold F. Schuknecht, chief of otolaryngology at the Massachusetts Eye and Ear Infirmary at Harvard.[15] Schuknecht was able to narrow down the possible sites of damage and to confirm that the vertigo arose from the posterior semicircular canal. He also correctly determined

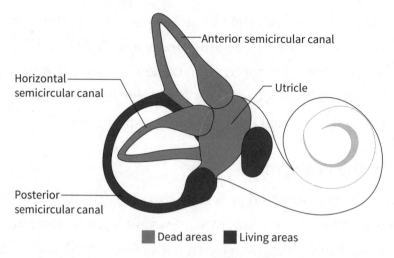

Figure 2.6   Posterior semicircular canal and saccule in Lindsay's patients. The utricle, anterior and horizontal semicircular canals could not have caused the repeated vertigo spells in the patients seen by Lindsay, because they were completely destroyed (light grey). Only the posterior semicircular canal and saccule (dark grey) remained intact and able to be the source of the patients' dizziness.

that the dizziness was set off by otoconia released from damaged utricles.

During his lifetime, Schuknecht collected temporal bones (the part of the skull containing the ear) from cadavers of people who had experienced dizziness. On studying specimens from two people with BPPV, he found deposits on the cupula of the posterior semicircular canal, which led him to believe that BPPV resulted from *cupulolithiasis*. Cupulolithiasis occurs when heavy particles—the otoconia— are stuck to the cupula, the spinning sensor located at one end of the semicircular canal. It was Schuknecht who believed that the weight of the particles makes the cupula heavy and causes attacks when a person lies down on one side (Figure 2.7). At that time, Schuknecht did not know what kind of material made up the particles, which were later identified as otoconia.

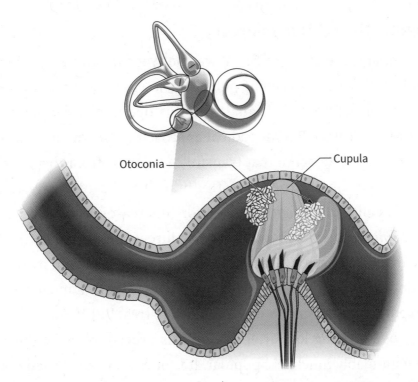

Otoconia   Cupula

Figure 2.7 Cupulolithiasis. The attachment of heavy particles (the otoconia) to the cupula was at first thought to cause the attacks of BPPV in people who are lying down. This theory did not explain why the spells are so brief, since heavy particles should keep the cupula deflected and the sensor turned on for as long as the person remains lying down.

In a paper published in 1969,[16] Schuknecht reasoned that these particles could be dispersed in the fluid that fills the inner ear, which was true. But he was not able to explain how free-floating particles could cause an attack without directly adhering to the cupula, so he proposed cupulolithiasis as the sole cause of BPPV. After this paper was published, most researchers believed that particles from the adjacent utricle were adherent to or impacting the cupula and this is what caused BPPV spells. This idea was ultimately proven wrong. It is still believed that cupulolithiasis happens in rare cases, but it is not the cause of most BPPV.

Singular Neurectomy Surgery

Even though the cause of BPPV was not yet fully understood when Schuknecht's work was being published, it was known that the problem was in the posterior canal, and this opened up the possibility of surgical treatment. One radical approach to treatment is surgery to disconnect the nerve that transmitted signals from the posterior semicircular canal to the brain. This branch of the inferior vestibular nerve is called the *singular nerve*; for this reason, the procedure is called *singular neurectomy*. This procedure was reported for the first time by Dr. Richard R. Gacek at Harvard in 1974[17,18] and its use has continued, although the need for such an invasive treatment declined markedly once exercises were developed to treat BPPV. Some patients developed hearing loss after having this procedure, which made it understandably much less popular. It is only very rarely used now in cases of BPPV that recur frequently and are severe.

Pistons and Plungers

The next major advance, and the one that was the most important to finding a simple treatment, was reported in 1979 paper by Drs. Stephen F. Hall, Ralph Ruby, and Joseph McClure, otolaryngologists at Queen's University and the University of Western Ontario in London, Ontario.[19] These three physicians effectively overturned the idea that the source of most BPPV was due to particles attached to the cupula of the posterior semicircular canal by showing that BPPV could be explained as resulting from dense particles moving in the fluid within the semicircular canal itself. Pistons and plungers are often used to move fluid in our daily lives. Think of how a plunger pulls the fluid in a narrow drainpipe of a sink back and forth until a clog is released. Or how a piston in a car cylinder moving up and down can pull gasoline into the engine. In BPPV, there is a clog of heavy ontoconia within the narrow tube of the semicircular canal. As this clog moves back and forth in the canal, it becomes a piston that pulls the fluid in the canal along with it. The sensor of the canal, the cupula, moves whenever the fluid moves, so this piston action turns the sensor "on" whenever gravity moves the heavy clump of otoconia. Hall, Ruby, and McClure reasoned that free-floating heavy crystals—which they correctly suspected were otoconia—in the long arm of the posterior semicircular canal were therefore responsible for the sudden vertigo attacks of BPPV.

This 1979 paper was key to finally understanding and treating the disorder. In a 1992 article, Drs. Lorne S. Parnes and Joseph McClure at the University of Western Ontario, the presence of the particles was directly confirmed and the particles were identified as degenerated otoconia.[20] The condition, which was ultimately called *canalithiasis* (meaning "stones in the canal"), is the most common cause of BPPV. It occurs when otoconia are moving freely within the semicircular canal, causing vertigo and nystagmus that resolves within 60 seconds (Figure 2.8 on the next page). The spells stop at the moment when the particles reach the lowest part of the canal and come to rest.

At this point, the reason for the attacks was finally clear. A sharp head movement, blow, or direct damage to the gravity-sensing utricle causes otoconia to be released into the fluids of the inner ear. If the otoconia enter the posterior semicircular canal in large enough numbers, they can clump together to form a piston, which causes movement in the fluids of the canal as the clog moves. This turns on the sensor by causing the cupula to move. As a result of this chain of events, BPPV symptoms occur. It is the movement of a clump of

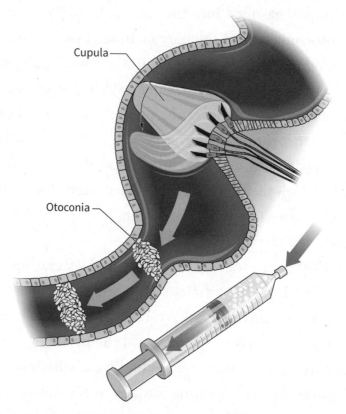

Cupula

Otoconia

Figure 2.8 Canalithiasis. A clot of heavy particles moving freely in the semicircular canal acts, just like a piston in a syringe does, to move the cupula. Gravity sets off movement of the particles, and they settle again once they reach the lowest part of the canal. This explains the short (merely seconds) duration of BPPV vertigo spells.

otoconia under the influence of gravity that sets off an attack. In BPPV, there are often many otoconia, sometimes many hundreds, forming one or several clumps in the canal.

Until 1980, the only exercise treatment for BPPV was the Cawthorne–Cooksey exercise program, but it took weeks for symptoms to resolve. That year, however, two new maneuvers were presented to the world.

The Brandt–Daroff Maneuver

In 1980, Dr. Thomas Brandt at the University of Munich and Dr. Robert Daroff, who was the Chairman of Neurology at Case Western Reserve University in Ohio, published an article about an exercise for treating BPPV.[21] This exercise, the *Brandt–Daroff maneuver*, is still used by some. The maneuver was, at the very least, an improvement on surgery for the condition. It improved on the program by Cawthorne because it eliminated all the Cawthorne–Cooksey exercises aimed at other vertigo diseases that were not useful for BPPV. The Brandt–Daroff exercise requires essentially performing the Dix–Hallpike maneuver over and over, first on one side and then on the other side. Although the head movements are exactly the same as the Dix–Hallpike, the Brandt–Daroff maneuver is done with the subject sitting on the side of the bed and falling to the side onto one shoulder, sitting back upright, and then falling onto the other shoulder, instead of sitting on a bed and lying straight backward as in the Dix–Hallpike. If particles are in the posterior semicircular canal, the Brandt–Daroff maneuver causes them to slosh about halfway around the canal toward the exit, so over time some particles gradually make their way one by one out of the canal. It can take days or weeks and many repetitions of the Brandt–Daroff maneuver to result in a resolution of symptoms, but for many patients this was far preferable to surgery.

The problem with the Brandt–Daroff maneuver was that patients had to endure the vertigo attacks the maneuver brought on, over and over for days or weeks, and many patients experienced only a very slow and gradual lessening of discomfort. People who didn't mind vertigo had always gotten better just from tossing their heads around anyway, so the Brandt–Daroff maneuver was not really that much of an advance for those people. At the same time, this maneuver was especially difficult for the people who needed relief the most: those who were afraid to move their heads out of fear of dizziness and so failed to resolve symptoms by natural head movements. Although this exercise is still sometimes recommended for BPPV, it is obsolete. Newer methods are much quicker and more effective.

A Quick and Effective Treatment at Last: The Epley Maneuver

Later in1980 at a professional meeting of ear surgeons, Dr. John Epley of Portland, Oregon, presented a technique that was based on the recently discovered information about free-floating particles. Epley reasoned that, since the canals are open on one end and the particles are floating freely, it should be possible to use gravity to draw the particles out of the posterior semicircular canal by placing the head in certain positions. Epley figured out a series of movements to rotate these particles out and end BPPV attacks in patients. Epley's series of movements begin with the Dix–Hallpike maneuver. After this, the patient rolls over onto the opposite side before sitting up (Figure 2.9).

Epley had performed his maneuver on several patients and found that it completely and quickly resolved the symptoms of the disease in a single treatment session. However, the treatment was so unusual that he could not convince his colleagues that it worked. A paper he wrote in 1983 was rejected and it took another nine years for a paper he wrote on the subject to be accepted and printed.[22]

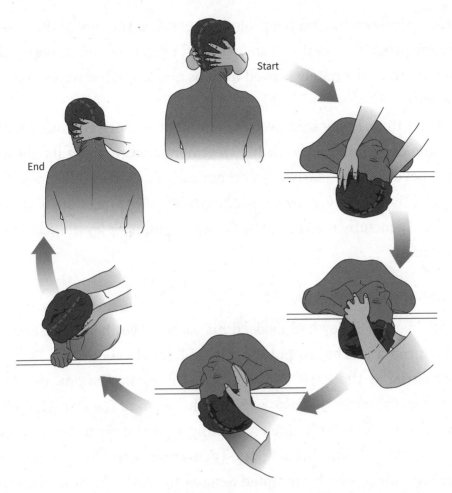

Figure 2.9   Epley maneuver. The patient lies down with the head turned, he or she then rolls to the opposite side and sits back up. This movement shifts the particles in the posterior semicircular canal toward the exit of the canal. In this example, the right ear is being treated.

During this time, rumors spread about this cure, but it remained controversial.[23] Physicians expect new treatments to involve medications or surgery. It was odd to hear about a treatment that was simply a series of head movements that had instant results. The extent of the rejection was surprising, however, as physicians had already fully embraced the prolonged physical therapy of the Cawthorne program and the Brandt–Daroff exercise, even though neither of these ultimately proved to be as quick or effective as Epley's exercise.

Over time, Epley won over the doubters as more and more physicians experimented with his treatment and realized its ability to relieve vertigo nearly instantaneously. Epley himself modestly named the maneuver the *canalith repositioning procedure* (CRP),[24] but it is generally referred to by the eponymous *Epley maneuver* in his honor.

The Semont Maneuver

In 1988, after Epley had devised his exercise but before he finally convinced a journal to publish his first article about it, a French physiatrist at the Paris Ear Institute, Dr. Alain Semont, devised another maneuver that also began with a form of the Dix–Hallpike maneuver.[25] Semont had been treating a patient with BPPV when the patient fell onto his side and then arose surprisingly cured of the symptoms, which prompted Semont to create the new exercise. Semont and his colleagues, Drs. G. Freyss and E. Vitte, proposed in their paper that they were treating cupulolithiasis (particles attached to the cupula) and that the brisk movements of their maneuver detached particles from the cupula and allowed the particles to exit through the canal. In Semont's maneuver, the patient sits on the side of the table. The clinician performs a Dix–Hallpike to the affected side, then has the patient sit back up and next lie down with the opposite shoulder down. This is very similar to the Brandt–Daroff maneuver. However, unlike in the Brandt–Daroff maneuver, Semont had the patient face the bed when lying on the opposite shoulder.

This small change made it easier for the particles to leave the semi-circular canal. Although Semont devised his maneuver to dislodge particles from the cupula,[26] his method worked to remove the free-floating particles that cause typical BPPV. During the years before Epley published his technique, this maneuver, named the *Semont maneuver* after its creator, became increasingly popular in Europe. This maneuver is discussed in more detail in Chapter 10, "Maneuvers Performed by a Provider."

Surgical Approaches to BPPV

In 1990 in Ontario, Parnes and McClure, who had, a decade before, first noted the loose-floating particles in the posterior semicircular canal in BPPV patients, came up with a new surgery to relieve the resulting symptoms.[27] The surgery involved plugging the semi-circular canal with bone that partitioned the canal so that fluid could no longer move and the loose particles could no longer set off vertigo. Unfortunately, although this surgery can be effective, hearing loss and balance problems are occasional side effects, as is the case with most surgeries that have been proposed to address BPPV. This surgery is still in limited use for very severe, recurrent cases of BPPV.

Because maneuvers do not have the serious side effects of surgeries and are so effective, very few people now undergo any type of surgery for BPPV. Surgery candidates are exclusively patients with intractable symptoms, such as people with a history of head trauma, those who experience very frequent recurrences, and patients who have crystals in multiple canals that keep re-entering. Sometimes, doctors employ destructive surgeries, such the destruction of the entire labyrinth: injecting the ear with medications that destroy vestibular function or severing the vestibular nerve. This is particularly true in cases that combine BPPV with other serious vertigo disorders.

Learning More about BPPV

After Epley finally published a description of his maneuver in 1992, the maneuver rapidly began to be used across the world. As use of the Epley maneuver spread, researchers began to notice that BPPV could affect all three semicircular canals and each location caused different symptoms of vertigo and required different maneuvers. Researcher also began to notice unexpected complications of some of the treatments. Although the major discoveries to date had outlined the cause of the disease and proposed effective ways to treat it, the medical community's knowledge of the disease was not yet complete. Since then, many new avenues of study have been explored. This book covers the key relevant points about the disorder that have become known since Epley paved the way to effective treatment with his simple and elegant maneuver.

As this chapter highlights, even though BPPV is a very simple mechanical disease, it took the work of many researchers around the world and several decades to understand the main features of BPPV and to develop an effective treatment. In the next chapter, the anatomy and mechanisms of BBPV are explained in more detail and show how and why the disorder strikes.

3

How Does Vertigo Happen?

Janet writes:

“My vertigo was so bad, I would fall to the floor. I joked that it was like having all the benefits of being drunk without all the calories, but in truth, it was not funny at all. My physician had given me medication and exercises that didn't work for me—I realized after your video it was because I didn't understand the spatial geometry of why we have to turn in the various directions. (The author's video can be viewed at the following link: https://tinyurl.com/kqa8u5s.) I suffered for two weeks, stumbling around like a crazy person before I found your video late Friday. I had to do your maneuver three or four times, but eventually the vertigo subsided, and I've had a weekend of no vertigo and I'm back to work this morning! I'm so grateful! Your simple explanation and the video of the girl doing the exercise solved the problem for me!”

People with benign posterior positional vertigo (BPPV) often come to my clinic saying they have loose crystals in their ears, but most don't really know why there are crystals in the ears, what makes them become loose, or how that makes the world appear to spin. In this chapter, we take a close look at the mechanics of vertigo.

BPPV and Spinning Vertigo

Almost everybody has experienced vertigo at some point in their lives. A toddler will start turning in a circle over and over and become fascinated by the strange sensation when they stop; older kids whirl on the playground at school and stagger off laughing. When you spin in place you see the environment turning around you and you might start to feel off balance. When you stop, the environment may reverse direction and spin crazily for several seconds even though you are no longer moving. This is a normal form of vertigo.

Vertigo is a sensation of movement, usually spinning, that is experienced when no movement is occurring. The inner ear is a motion sensor that can detect spinning or turning in any direction. The inner ear is also responsible for our ability to feel the pull of gravity and the sensation of accelerating in a straight line.

We can add adjectives in front of the word vertigo to better explain the various feelings people experience when they have vertigo. *Spinning vertigo* describes the illusion of circular motion; *elevator vertigo* refers to a feeling of vertical dropping or rising; *rocking vertigo* is a sense of rocking as if on a boat; *tilt vertigo* makes it feel as though the world is tilting and gravity is pulling from an unexpected direction; and *linear vertigo* is experienced as a false sense of acceleration or deceleration forward or back, like you might feel riding in a fast car. When the inner ear malfunctions, any of these forms of vertigo can occur.

BPPV only causes spinning vertigo. All the other forms of vertigo described in the previous paragraph arise from the gravity sensors of the inner ear (see p. 16 and Figure 2.3) and we will discuss these forms further in Chapter 4, "Non-BPPV Causes of Vertigo." None of the other forms (elevator, rocking, tilt, or linear vertigo) are experienced by people who only have BPPV.

Spinning sensations arise from the semicircular canals, and this discovery was the tip-off that led to the realization that BPPV is a semicircular canal disease and can be cured very simply (see Chapter 2 , "The History of Benign Paroxysmal Positional Vertigo (BPPV)," for more on the history of the disorder and its treatments).

The Evolution of Human Motion Sensors

How did humans come to be so sensitive to vertigo in all its forms? Since spinning sensors can cause vertigo, it might seem pointless to have them when people really don't spin around very often. Like so many other parts of the body, however, spinning sensors are very important in ways that are easy to overlook. The spinning sensors are used every time the head is moved, because every head movement requires a small head rotation. The sensors link to balance reflexes that prevent falling, and to eye reflexes that keep vision from blurring. It has taken millions of years to refine our spinning sensors to perform these functions to perfection.

Being able to sense movement and orientation is critical for creatures that need to move about their environment, and primitive motion sensors were already present in animals 500 million years ago. These early motion sensors allowed swimming animals to feel the effect of gravity, allowing them to distinguish up from down and to feel tilt. Two hundred million years later, a more sophisticated spinning sensor developed in some animals. All animals with semicircular canals, including humans, descend from the animals who first were able to sense spinning and rotation.

Hundreds of millions of years ago, all animals lived in water, and being able to sense the flow of water over the body was a useful skill. To enable this, the *hair cell* evolved. Hair cells have many fine hairs, called *cilia* (singular: *cilium*), that look like the fibers of a paint brush sticking up from the cell (Figure 3.1). Just as the hairs of a paint brush bend to the side as the brush is dragged through paint, a hair cell's cilia bend as the cell moves.

In order for the hair cell to serve as a useful motion sensor, an animal needed to have some way of communicating this bending of cilia to the brain. In addition, it was important to know which direction the cilia were tilting and how quickly this was happening. Each hair cell has rows of cilia arranged in a series of stairsteps from shortest to tallest, with a specialized tall and thick knobbed cilium at the very back. The tip of each cilia is attached to the side of the taller one next to it, so the movement of any cilia helps drag along the neighbors, all in the same direction. When the hairs all move toward the tallest and thickest cilium (the one with the ball on top in Figure 3.1) at the back of the

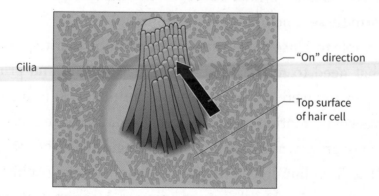

Figure 3.1 Hair cell and its cilia. Every cell has this characteristic stairstep arrangement of hair-like cilia. The hair with a ball on top is the thickest and when the cilia are swept in this direction, this turns "on" the cell.

tallest row, the signal to the brain switches ON, and when the hairs all move towards the shortest cilia, the signal is in the OFF direction.[1]

Hair cells like these arranged along the outside of the body in swimming animals made it possible for our early animal ancestors to pick up water movement in any direction. By summing the impulses from many hair cells, a sense of the strength or speed of the movement could also be detected. This was how early animals gradually developed a three-dimensional sense of the movement of water.

The Gravity Sensors

Feeling the movement of water outside the body helped marine animals know they were in motion but feeling the movement of the head would prove to be even more useful. The first motion sensor inside the head was a gravity sensor. An ability to detect gravity comes in handy, for example, if an animal wants to attach itself to the ocean floor with its head up, rather than ending up upside down. A sense of gravity also helps animals move up in the ocean to shallower waters where sunlight is more plentiful and it is warm, rather than down toward darker and colder waters. A gravity sensor requires something relatively heavy in the head. If a heavy object is present, then when gravity pulls down on this heavy object, hair cells can sense the direction of pull. Some animals solved the need for a heavy object by allowing small rocks or sand to enter their inner ears. Higher animals including humans, "grow" their own rocks in the form of calcium carbonate crystals called *otoconia*. Calcium carbonate is the same thing as chalk powder. Like chalk, it is white and forms crystals. The key thing about calcium carbonate is that it is more dense than the fluid

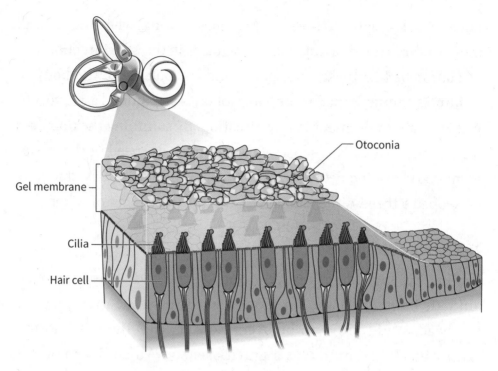

Figure 3.2 The gravity sensor. Hair cells of this sensor have bundles of cilia projecting into a sticky gel layer with the otoconia crystals piled on top. As the head tilts, the crystals shift, indicating a change in the direction of gravity.

inside the inner ear, so it sinks down to the lowest part of the ear under the influence of gravity.

In modern humans, the otoconial calcium carbonate crystals are piled up on top of a gel membrane that covers thousands of hair cells (Figure 3.2), and it is the shifting of this pile of crystals that tells us when our heads are upright or tilted, and whether we are accelerating in a line and in which direction that acceleration is happening.[2] The crystals are covered with a sticky substance that helps them stay in place, but they can be knocked loose if the head is hit hard enough, or if the head is accelerated or decelerated in a sudden jerky fashion as it can be, for example, during amusement park rides.

The Spinning Sensors

It was only after gravity sensors arose in our ancestors that a turning motion sensor inside the inner ear developed. The motion sensor consists of hair cells whose cilia stretch like a fan across a round fluid-filled chamber (Figure 3.3). The hair cells are embedded in a sticky gel that serves to bind the cilia from thousands of hair cells into a single structure. The round chamber is attached to a circular tube and the opening of the tube faces the fan of cilia at a 90-degree

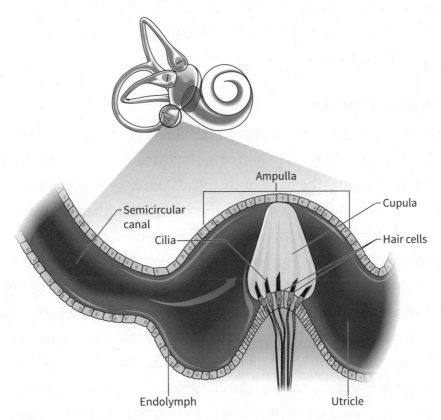

Figure 3.3 The spinning sensor. The cilia on top of the hair cells project into a gel to form the cupula, which stretches across the ampulla like a partition. When a person turns, the fluid in the semicircular canal (the endolymph) moves the cupula, bending the cilia and turning the sensor on or off.

angle. The tube serves to direct any fluid moving through the tube straight at the center of the fan of cells. The tube is the semicircular canal, the round chamber is the ampulla, and the fan of cells is the cupula. Once semicircular canals developed, humans and other mammals had three semicircular canals in each ear and became able to feel movement in three dimensions.

Humans ultimately evolved to have an inner ear divided between hearing and balance. Each ear has five motion sensors: two gravity sensors containing crystals and three spinning sensors that pick up fluid movement in the semicircular canals. All the sensors are filled with the same fluid, and that fluid moves through and connects all the motion sensors together.

The Semicircular Canals

The terminology for the semicircular canals can be confusing. In all animal species other than humans, the three canals are named the posterior (toward the back of the head), anterior (toward the front of the head), and horizontal (in the horizontal plane of the head) semicircular canals. In human surgical anatomy, these same canals are given new names: The posterior canal is called *inferior* (lowest in the head); the anterior canal is called *superior* (highest in the head), and the horizontal canal is called *lateral* (to the side in the head). Having these names helped surgeons recognize the canals as they were encountered in the skull while drilling. Over the years, the distinction between these two sets of names has lessened. Often these names are mixed up randomly, even in textbooks. BPPV is usually said to involve the posterior semicircular canal, for example, rather than the inferior canal. To give some consistency, in this book we use

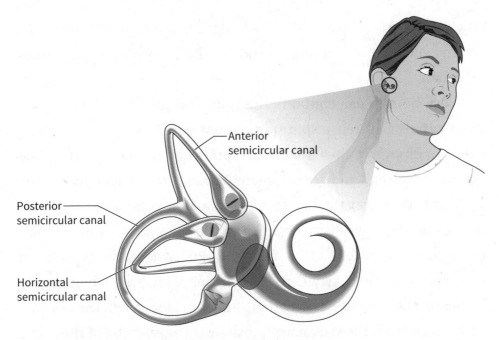

Anterior
semicircular canal

Posterior
semicircular canal

Horizontal
semicircular canal

Figure 3.4   The semicircular canals of the inner ear are named according to
their position in the head: anterior (toward the forehead), posterior (toward the
back of the head) and horizontal (in the horizontal plane).

the old animal nomenclature so we will talk only about the posterior,
anterior, and horizontal semicircular canals (Figure 3.4).

When Motion Sensors Malfunction

All our motion sensors have the capacity to malfunction. Even
though evolution works to gradually refine and improve the sensors
in our ears, because creatures find new ways to use their sensors over
time, there is always more work for evolution to do. When a sensor's
abilities don't match the organism's needs perfectly enough, problems can result. This is what happens in the inner ears of people with
BPPV. For people with BPPV, the crystals that are supposed to be

stuck to the gravity sensors instead migrate randomly around in the ear and end up in a spinning sensor, usually the posterior semicircular canal.

Every human ear contains the same design flaw. The semicircular canals that sense spinning are not complete circles. Instead they are circular tubes filled with fluid that are closed off by the sensor on one end and are completely open at the other end. On the open end, they are attached to a large cavity containing the utricle (one of our two gravity sensors), and the piles of otoconia resting on top of the utricle. As long as the head is upright, the crystals on the gravity sensor stay where they belong. However, when people lie flat on their backs or hang their heads upside down, the crystals can detach from the sensor and slosh near the opening of the semicircular canals. The crystals can move about in this way because the entire inner ear is filled with the same fluid, and the crystals can move anywhere along these fluid pathways (Figure 3.5). The openings that lead into all of the semicircular canals are just above the utricle and its otoconia when the head is upright, but when the head is upside down, this means the openings are right below this heavy pile of crystals. When the head is tipped back or upside down, if the crystals begin to slosh around and come off the sensor, it is quite easy for them to fall into the semicircular canals. Once the crystals fall into a semicircular canal and make it halfway around the ring of the canal, they are nearly past the point of no return. If a person then brings his or her head upright, gravity readily pulls the crystals all the way down into the bottom of the posterior canal. They are too heavy to jump back up and out from that location, and from that point on the person has BPPV.

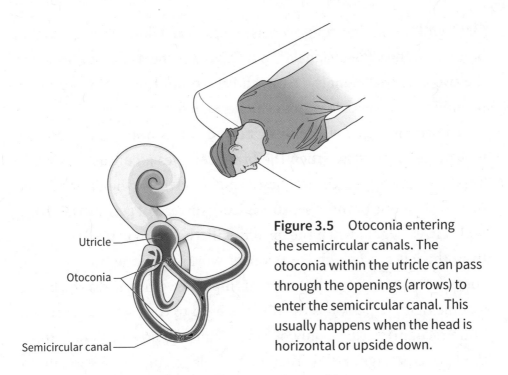

Figure 3.5 Otoconia entering the semicircular canals. The otoconia within the utricle can pass through the openings (arrows) to enter the semicircular canal. This usually happens when the head is horizontal or upside down.

Motion Sensors and Vertigo

There are two basic causes of vertigo: (1) turning *off* or losing one or more sensors, or (2) turning *on* one or more sensors when they should be *off*. To understand the difference, we need to discuss how the brain senses motion and interprets the signals our ears send.

The brain senses motion by perceiving and summing up electrical signals from both inner ears, and these should match perfectly. For example, when a person is not moving, the ears both signal with a low but steady stream of impulses. The brain interprets these signals to mean, "The ears are both the same; therefore, I am in NEUTRAL, not turning."

If a person turns his or her head to the right, the semicircular canals in the right ear increase the flow of signals which tells the brain "I am

ON," while a simultaneous decrease in the usual flow of signals to the brain from the left ear signals "I am OFF." It is the difference between the two ears that signals a turn, and the brain thinks the person is turning toward the side with the higher signal flow.

If a person's ear is suddenly destroyed, for example, if the left ear is damaged by a virus, then the brain receives a confusing signal. This is what happens in the first type of vertigo (when a sensor is turned *off* or one or more sensors is lost). Instead of getting the "I am NEUTRAL" signal when the head is still, the brain gets "I am OFF" from the left ear (which is no longer working) while the right ear continues to give a small stream of impulses. This makes the brain assume that the person is turning the head to the right, because the brain recognizes turns only by comparing the flow of signals from the two ears (Figure 3.6). The brain "feels" a turn even though no turn is occurring, and this is experienced as vertigo.

The acceleration of a turn is determined by the strength of the signal each ear sends. Imagine a sensor can send any amount of signals per second on a scale of 1 to 10. The resting, neutral state is about 2 in both ears, which the brain sees as a right turn of 2 and a left turn of 2, so they cancel each other out. When a person makes a very fast accelerating turn to the right, like whipping the head around to the right after hearing a gunshot, the signals may increase up to 8 or 9 in the right ear. At the same time, the signals from the left ear drop from 2 to 0. The brain interprets the difference of 8 or 9 points on the scale as a very intense right turn or spinning.

If there is no turn happening, but the left ear shuts off because it is injured, this causes a false sense of rotation or vertigo. The left

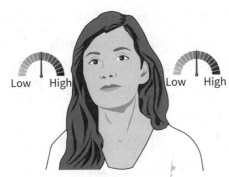

1. Not moving

Both ears working

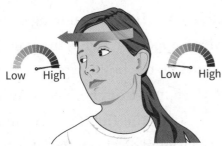

2. Right head turn

Both ears working

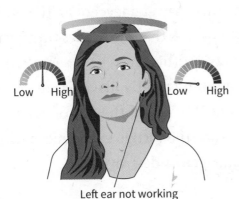

3. Vertigo

Left ear not working

Figure 3.6 Electric signals during head turns. (1) Normal, not moving: Both ears have a low steady flow of signals. (2) Normal head turn: When the head turns right, the number of signals increase from the right ear and decrease from the left, and you feel a right turning sensation. (3) Vertigo: If the left ear stops working because of damage, even though the head is not moving, signals continue from the right ear but decrease from the left ear. This is felt as a turn to the right and is the reason vertigo makes you feel like you are spinning.

ear goes from its resting state of 2 to 0 but the right ear continues to be at 2, so the feeling of acceleration and vertigo is only at 2, not very extreme compared to a quick head turn. The person then feels a continuous but slow right turn, rather like the turn you make when tracking a person walking across a room.

Let's look at the second cause of vertigo mentioned above—the vertigo caused by turning a sensor on when it should be off. In people with healthy ears, fluid always moves in the semicircular canals of both ears at the same time. It usually moves in opposite directions in two canals, so they cancel each other out. If fluid is moving in only one semicircular canal, which is what happens in BPPV, then vertigo can occur. When the head is not moving, the brain expects to pick up constant, slow, steady NEUTRAL signals from both ears. When fluid moves in only one horizontal canal (the right, for example), then the brain receives the NEUTRAL signal of 2 from the left canal, while the stimulated right canal signals "I am ON" and provides the acceleration and direction of the turn, say at a level of 8. The brain sums all this information up and assumes that the head is turning to the right at an acceleration of $8 - 2 = 6$. This creates the sensation of vertigo, and the sensation is of spinning tightly like a figure skater. This is the problem that occurs in BPPV, and the reason why the vertigo of BPPV is much stronger than the vertigo experienced when an ear or semicircular canal is damaged or destroyed.

Eyes and Ears: Vision and Vertigo

It isn't only the brain that feels spinning when vertigo occurs. If the spinning sensation is fast enough, you can actually see the world spinning around you. This happens because controlling eye movements is one of the most important functions of the inner ears. When you're watching a video, it's very noticeable when the camera is jiggled or pans too quickly. The picture becomes a messy blur that can even be a little nauseating to watch. When making a video recording, it is important to move very slowly and hold the camera steadily to prevent this. If there were no inner ears, all vision would look like a jumpy video.

The inner ear prevents the images we see from jiggling even when we move quickly. It does this through a very fast reflex, the fastest in the whole body. This reflex is called the *vestibulo-ocular reflex* because it passes between the inner ear (the vestibular system) and the eyes (*oculus* in Latin). Part of the reason the eyes and ears are located close together in the head is so that the path for these reflexes can be very short, making the reflex extremely quick.

Here is an experiment you can do to test your reflexes. Pick a word on the page to look at. Look at that word and turn your head from side to side or up and down, gradually speeding up. If your ears are functioning normally, you should be able to keep that word in focus even when turning or jiggling your head very quickly. The word should not start shifting or jerking back and forth.

Every time your head turns to the right, your inner ears sense the turn and send information to the centers in your brainstem that control eye movements. This causes the eye to turn in the exact opposite direction from the head turn at exactly the same speed and acceleration as the head is turning, so the net effect is that the eyes stay in the same place in space. If you want to check this, look at your eyes in a mirror while you turn your head. You'll see the image of your eyes stay locked on yours even though your head is turning. It's as though your eyes are left behind every time you turn your head. This means that whatever you happen to be looking at stays in focus even though your head is moving. In this way, the inner ear steadies your vision.

What happens if you keep turning in a spin? Your eyes turn until they are stopped by reaching the corner of your lids and then they get dragged, just like a bad video. To prevent this, when you turn your head in a circle, your eyes move in the opposite direction of your head until the corner of the eye is reached, then jump quickly ahead, then again move to the corner, then jump quickly again. This slow rotation followed by a fast correction is called *nystagmus*. It is perfectly normal for nystagmus to happen when you are making a big rotation of your head and body, but should never happen when you are not moving.

When you have vertigo, the brain thinks it is turning continuously, so it sends the eye moving in this jerking, repeating pattern. If someone looks at the eyes of a person who is very dizzy, they may be able to see nystagmus—the slow-one-way, fast-in-the-other-way jerking of the eyes. The direction that the eyes jerk is related to the direction of the feeling of vertigo the person is experiencing. It can be side to side, up and down, or even at an angle. In *torsional* nystagmus, the eyes actually rotate on their stalks and the pupils seem to jump clockwise or counterclockwise.

Now, let's return to discussing vertigo that occurs if a single semicircular canal is turned ON. Can we tell by looking at the eyes which canal is being turned on? The answer is yes. Imagine that we had X-ray vision and could look right through the eyes and through the skull to look at the semicircular canals. When the eye is centered and facing forward, the direction that the eye moves with stimulation of one canal is a projection of that semicircular canal (Figure 3.7) onto the eye.[3,4]

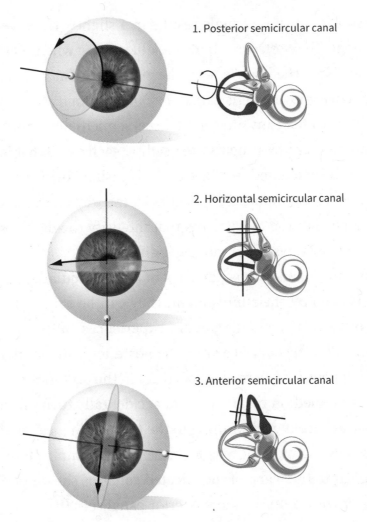

1. Posterior semicircular canal

2. Horizontal semicircular canal

3. Anterior semicircular canal

Figure 3.7 Nystagmus eye movements caused by problems in the semicircular canals. (1) When the posterior canal (dark grey) is stimulated, the eyes will both move in a circular direction. (2) When the horizontal canal (dark grey) is stimulated, the eyes move from side to side. (3) When the anterior canal (dark grey) is stimulated, the eyes move up and down at a slight tilt.

That means that if the problem is in the *horizontal* canals, which look pretty much like a horizontal line when seen from the front of the head, the eyes go back and forth in a horizontal line during nystagmus. The *anterior* canals look mostly like a tilted vertical line, and so a problem in these canals results in a slightly tilted vertical eye movement. The *posterior* canals look like a ring when seen from the front, and so if the issue is here, the eye movement is more circular. This circular movement is called *torsional nystagmus*.

BPPV can affect any one (or all three) semicircular canals in either ear, and different treatments are used for each canal that is affected. This will be discussed in Chapter 9, "Unusual Forms of BPPV." No matter which canal the BPPV occurs in, the way vertigo is generated is the same, but the movements that intensify the dizziness are different and the ways of diagnosing it differ also.

Any time a person has particles in a semicircular canal that can cause vertigo by their movement, they can be said to have BPPV. Most of the time, when a person experiences BPPV, the particles are located in the curved arm of the posterior semicircular canal. If BPPV happens when a mass of particles in the posterior semicircular canal are pulled on by gravity and accidentally turn on that canal, this causes a feeling of spinning in the plane of that canal and causes torsional nystagmus. The axis of the perceived spinning is exactly perpendicular to the plane of the affected canal, as shown in Figure 3.7. A person with BPPV in the posterior canal sees the room spin in a circle upward in a spiral and tilted to one side. The faster the feeling of vertigo, the faster the jerking of the eyes in nystagmus. BPPV is one of the fastest forms of vertigo that a person can feel, so to an observer the eyes can look like they are whirling violently in their sockets. The torsional nystagmus tends to start slowly, builds rapidly to a peak over a few seconds, and then slows down until it stops, all over the course of a few seconds.

Crystals and Vertigo

The vertigo of BPPV can range from mild, momentary dizziness to extremely violent and more prolonged spells lasting up to a minute. The reason for the variability has to do with how many otoconia crystals are in motion. A few crystals that do not form any clumps in the semicircular canals are not enough to cause any symptoms. Once a clump forms, larger numbers of crystals increases the mass of the clump, and that translates into more piston power.[5] The larger the piston, the stronger the movement of the cupula and the more intense the spinning becomes. The length of time the spinning is felt is determined by the mass of crystals and how far along the semicircular canal they travel. Just jiggling a mass of particles causes only a moment of spinning. In contrast, flipping the head upside down allows the particles to move slowly around half the circumference of the semicircular canal, prolonging the spinning, which may last for half a minute or more.

Does the posterior canal still work when crystals are stuck in it? Even though crystals are present, head movements that normally stimulate the posterior canal still cause normal responses of the eyes. When the head is turned, the crystals move along in the fluid at the same speed as the fluid moves in the canal. You can't tell they are there. However, after the head movement stops and the fluid should have stopped moving, in BPPV the eyes continue to move. If the particles fall because gravity is pulling them to the lowest part of the canal, the clump of otoconia collectively acts as a piston and drags fluid away from the cupula and the signal the brain receives is of continued movement. The eyes continue to move because the fluid is being moved by this piston effect. It is then that you see the world appear to spin.

As we noted earlier, BPPV can affect any one (or all three) semi-circular canals and different treatments are used for each canal. The movement that most precisely stimulates the posterior canal on the right side is when the head is turned 45 degrees toward the right shoulder and tilted upward looking over the shoulder towards the sky (Figure 3.8). This movement rotates the head almost exactly in the plane of that semicircular canal. The Dix–Hallpike maneuver (discussed on pp. 20–23) also rotates the head in the plane of the canal, but moves the head from upright all the way around until it is almost hanging upside down. This means any particles in the canal

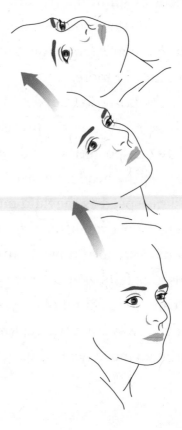

Figure 3.8 Head movement to stimulate the posterior canal. The head is turned 45 degrees to the right. As the head is lifted from this position, the posterior canal is rotated in the plane of the head movement. This moves the fluid in the canal.

have to move a long distance around the canal as gravity pulls on them, maximizing the duration of the nystagmus and so making the nystagmus easier for the practitioner to observe. The Dix–Hallpike maneuver also has another benefit: It moves the particles in the direction of the exit from the canal, so by the time the nystagmus stops, the particles are nearly half of the way out of the canal.

Vertigo can come from many causes other than BPPV, but only BPPV responds to maneuvers. The different causes of vertigo can be diagnosed by examining the type of spinning or movement sensations that occur, what sets off spells, how long the attacks last, and other characteristics. The next chapter discusses the kinds of vertigo that do not respond to BPPV maneuvers.

4

Non-BPPV Causes of Vertigo

"Anna was a thirty-five-year-old woman who tended to get motion sickness. She experienced it when riding in the car on mountain roads, and also when boating if the water was rough. She also experienced migraines—throbbing headaches on one side of her head that made her feel nauseated and dizzy. Sometimes there would be a crinkling, shimmering rainbow in her vision that could make it difficult to see for 15 minutes or so. This was usually followed by a bad headache. One day during a headache, Anna noticed a low, humming sound in her left ear. She also noticed her hearing seemed obstructed. About an hour later, the room began to slowly spin, and the feeling got worse if Anna moved her head at all. All of this set off her motion sickness and she vomited a couple of times. After about three hours, the spinning and ringing began to diminish. A few months later, the whole thing happened again. These repeated spells became a new, unwelcome aspect of Anna's life."

In Chapter 3, "How Does Vertigo Happen?" we discussed classic spinning vertigo, the type of vertigo caused by benign paroxysmal positional vertigo (BPPV). But BPPV is not the only condition that results in vertigo. There are many other causes for vertigo. Because all the treatments that have been devised for BPPV only work for vertigo induced by BPPV, and are not helpful for any other kind, it is important to know the difference. This chapter discusses vertigo that is not caused by BPPV.

Recall from Chapter 3, "How Does Vertigo Happen?" that the two basic causes for inner ear vertigo are (1) turning off or losing one or more sensors or (2) turning on one or more sensors when they should be off. Some diseases cause vertigo for the first reason—they shut off sensors for short periods of time. These periods are generally followed by recovery but gradual damage can accumulate from the repeated spells caused by these diseases over time. In other diseases that cause vertigo for the same reason (sensors that are mistakenly turned off), the sensors remain intact even after many years of spells. Diseases that cause vertigo for the second reason—inappropriately stimulated sensors that are on when they should be off such as BPPV, for example, do not usually result in damage to the sensors.

Sensor Damage: The Loss of One or More Spinning Sensors

As this chapter discusses vertigo that is not caused by BPPV, here we are primarily discussing the first cause of vertigo—vertigo that results when one or more inner ear sensors turn off when they should be on. Sensor damage is one of the most common reasons vertigo occurs. It may happen when the nerve leading to the sensor is injured, blood flow to the sensors or their nerves is stopped or restricted, or the hair cells stop working. If the entire sensor is destroyed, the onset of vertigo is immediate and the environment usually spins for a few days (see Chapter 3, "How Does Vertigo Happen?" for the reason this starts). This often sets off vomiting that is made worse by sudden head movement. The vertigo gradually lessens as the days pass and becomes tolerable after about a week. Sometimes recovery is more gradual and can take months to a year or more. The more sensors that are involved and the greater the injury to each sensor, the worse the vertigo is and the more prolonged the recovery is. When an inner ear is completely destroyed, some symptoms of dizziness may linger for years afterward. (See Figure 3.6 and pp. 35–48 for a more detailed discussion of what happens when a sensor is turned off.) As time goes by, the brain learns to pay less attention to the sensors and rebalances the signals so the spinning gradually declines.

Each of these health issues can have slightly different symptoms, but all can cause repeated dizzy spells. The differences between the spells of these diseases and BPPV are usually very clear. The damaging spells usually last much longer than BPPV. In BPPV, the actual spinning of the room lasts less than a minute, while in damaging disorders it can last many minutes to hours. Also, spells that are not caused by BPPV are not caused by making a simple head movement. Dizziness from these other non-BPPV causes come on all by themselves, without much warning.

There are many ways for sensors to be "turned off." A virus can cause swelling in the nerve leading to an ear, causing vestibular neuritis;[1] a head injury with a skull fracture can cut the nerve to the ear or directly damage the inner ear itself;[2] a stroke can cut off blood flow to an entire ear or portions of it (sudden sensorineural hearing loss);[3] or a drug that is toxic to the ear can injure the hair cells (ototoxicity; aminoglycosides, a type of antibiotic, are well known for causing ototoxicity).[4]

Different problems cause different kinds of vertigo episodes. Drugs, for example, tend to affect both ears when they cause ototoxicity. And if both are affected at the same time, a spinning feeling does not always result. Instead, these drugs tend to cause a gradual loss of balance while walking and blurred vision. When the ear is suddenly damaged by a virus and a person experiences vestibular neuritis, they experience a characteristic pattern of dizziness. It begins with severe dizziness that peaks in the first day or so. The dizziness diminishes gradually over a week to a much lower level, and then tapers off very slowly over many months. This kind of dizziness typically does not flare up again.

Causes of Vertigo That Result in Spinning Sensor Damage

In addition to viruses, injuries, medications, and malformation, there are also many kinds of diseases that cause repeated spells of dizziness. Some of these illnesses damage the ear, resulting in a gradual loss of hearing or balance function. Other illnesses cause equally intense spells, but the ear does not become damaged, so it can be hard to tell diseases like these apart at first.

Meniere's Disease

One of the most feared illnesses that causes dizziness is Meniere's disease.[5] This is the problem that Anna—the person described at the beginning of the chapter—has. Meniere's disease is a progressive, damaging disorder of the ear. Calling it a disease is a misnomer. It is really a collection of different problems all of which result in similar symptoms. The distinguishing characteristic of Meniere's disease affects the inner ears. People with Meniere's disease have an anatomical problem in the inner ears that can worsen over time. The inner ear is a very delicate, fluid-filled, and complicated structure

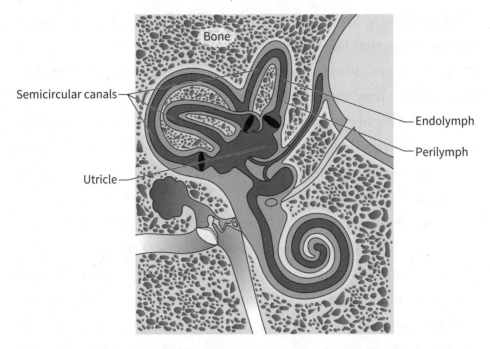

Figure 4.1 The fluids of the inner ear. The tubes and sacs that make up the inner ear are filled with fluid called endolymph (dark grey). Outside the membranes another fluid—perilymph (light grey)—cushions the inner ear from the bone that surrounds it.

that is separated from the bone surrounding it in the skull by a cushioning fluid called perilymph (Figure 4.1). In people with Meniere's disease, the amount of fluid inside the membrane in the inner ear begins to increase, causing the inner ear membrane to balloon and enlarge until it compresses or nearly fills the perilymph space. As a result, less cushioning is provided by the fluid surrounding the inner ear. This state is called endolymphatic hydrops, and when it occurs the ear becomes much more vulnerable to damage. The inner ear has difficulty regulating blood flow when endolymphatic hydrops is present and if the person with Meniere's disease has other health problems that reduce blood flow in the head, blood flow to the ear can fall so low that the ear shuts off temporarily.[6]

Different people can have very different reasons for experiencing low blood flow. One might have spasm in the arteries because of migraines; another may suffer from sleep apnea, and a third might have blood that does not clot properly. All of these Meniere's patients can end up with very similar attacks of vertigo, but the treatment for each will be somewhat different.

Spells of Meniere's disease last much longer than those of BPPV. A bad Meniere's spell might cause the room to appear to spin for 20 minutes; another might cause spinning that continues for several hours. A Meniere's sufferer may vomit over and over during an attack, and usually has to lie down and wait for it to pass. During these spells, the ear that has endolymphatic hydrops may feel constantly stuffy. A patient may also hear a sound in the ear, like the roaring of a vacuum cleaner. Hearing can diminish. Once the spell of spinning ends, though, the ear at first seems to have fully recovered. Over time, however, testing may reveal a slow, gradual loss of hearing and balance function. Eventually the ear can lose all serviceable hearing.

Other Problems That Can Damage Ear Spinning Sensors

Sometimes a cause of vertigo can be inherited. For instance, the inner ear can be congenitally malformed in such a way that causes vertigo.[7] Diseases in which the immune system begins to attack the person's own body by mistake can also result in damage to the ear sensors.[8]

Causes of Vertigo That Do Not Result in Sensor Damage

Vertigo can occur for a number of other reasons, and some of these causes of vertigo leave the inner ear sensors undamaged.

Dizziness and Migraine Headaches

BPPV causes spells of spinning over and over, but the ear goes on functioning normally in between spells. There are other diseases that can do the same thing. For example, people with migraines are prone to vertigo spells that can repeat for months or years without any damage detected in the ears.

The term vestibular migraine refers to dizziness in people who also experience migraine headaches.[9] There are many other names for this disorder, including migraine-associated dizziness, migraine-related vestibulopathy, and benign recurrent vertigo. Migraine headaches are a very common ailment that is most prevalent and severe in people who are between the ages of 12 and 50. It tends to affect women more than men, begins around puberty, and generally subsides after menopause in women. People with this condition usually develop severe migraine headaches or optical auras at some point in their lives. The classic migraine headache is a pounding, nauseating headache that goes on for hours. Lights can seem too intense, and even ordinary sounds can seem too loud during the headache, so a person with this problem will often go to bed in a darkened room and try to sleep off the headache.

Some people who experience migraines have more trouble with the aura than head pain.[10] Usually the aura is a visual problem in which a person sees a sparkling, rainbow-colored, curved zigzag of light that can last for minutes. Vision is dimmed or there can be a blind spot inside the curve. If either migraine headaches or auras are present, the person is at risk to experience dizzy spells. However, the dizziness can also come on completely separate from the headaches or aura—even years apart.

The dizzy spells migraine sufferers report are quite different from BPPV. BPPV spells are all nearly the same. In migraine, the spells differ from attack to attack. Sometimes the patient feels dizzy for a few minutes, and other times the dizziness goes on for days. Migraine patients may sometimes feel as though the room is shifting around them, and at other times they may feel as though the spinning is inside the head while the surrounding environment appears to be stable. Nausea is very common with these types of spells. While BPPV spells are set off by movements, the spells of migraine sufferers are more likely to be set off by eating certain foods, such as MSG (monosodium glutamate), chocolate, or red wine. Sometimes weather changes trigger dizziness for people who get migraines.

People with migraines are more prone to all dizziness than other people,[11] and migraines are also linked to Meniere's disease and BPPV. Many people with Meniere's disease have migrainous blood vessel spasm that result in low blood flow, but it is the endolymphatic hydrops that turns this into a damaging disorder. Migraine is inherited, so it is possible that entire families have similar dizziness problems. There are several medicines that help to prevent migraine headaches that can also be used to prevent the dizziness.

BPPV can be more common in people who have migraines and is also frequent in ears affected by Meniere's disease. People who have BPPV in addition to another vertigo disorder can still get relief from positional vertigo by doing the Half Somersault maneuver, but any dizziness caused by migraine or Meniere's will not be changed by maneuvers.

Dizziness and Sleep Apnea

Another common reason for repeated but reversible dizzy spells is sleep apnea.[12] Sleep apnea is a breathing problem that occurs while sufferers are sleeping at night and is associated with loud snoring, gasping or pauses in breathing while asleep, and frequent awakenings during the night. Having many momentary spells of vertigo throughout the day is typical for people with this disorder, but longer spells can also occur. Sleep apnea is common in people with Meniere's disease.

There are several other disorders that cause repeated dizzy spells that are harmless to the ear but can cause significant disability.

Dizziness Caused by Malfunctioning Gravity Sensors

Vertigo is a spinning feeling and this usually originates from the spinning sensors, the semicircular canals. However, recall from Chapter 2, "The History of BPPV," that each ear also has two gravity sensors. These gravity sensors can also malfunction. The sensations this damage can create can seem very bizarre. For example, it is possible for patients to experience a sudden rocking or tilting sensation.[13] The ground can appear to abruptly tilt up at an odd angle. People with malfunctioning gravity sensors may suddenly crash to the floor, feeling as if they were pushed. It can feel as if the floor has dropped out from under you like a falling elevator.

Malfunctioning gravity sensors cannot create the spinning sensation of BPPV. However, a virus that affects the inner ear, as discussed at the beginning of the chapter, can damage one or both gravity sensors. Sometimes this can cause otoconia, or heavy crystals, to be released from the sensor. If some of the semicircular canals in the damaged ear still have function, the released crystals can migrate into the canals and this can cause severe BPPV symptoms. Fortunately, like any other BPPV, this problem does respond to maneuvers.

In this chapter, we discussed non-BPPV causes of vertigo that are not caused by crystals moving in the canals and that cannot be improved with maneuvers. In the next chapter, we will introduce some types of positional dizziness that mimic BPPV but have their source in the brain itself (not the inner ears). These central nervous system disorders are often mistaken for BPPV but do not respond to BPPV treatment maneuvers.

5

Central Vertigo: Non-BPPV Positional Vertigo and Nystagmus

" Eduardo, a retired engineer, noticed that his balance was failing. He felt like he was staggering when he was walking and he was sometimes dizzy. Even more worrisome, he felt like he was flipping over forward when he lay down; this began to happen almost every time he reclined. By trial and error, he figured out that the problem was not as severe when he kept his head propped up so he raised the head of his adjustable bed so that he was almost sitting upright to sleep. Eduardo searched his symptoms online and found out about BPPV maneuvers. He tried them and experienced some mild vertigo during the maneuvers. Afterwards, the dizziness had not changed and his balance was still problematic. His coordination was affected; his hands trembled and his writing became hard to read. A physician Eduardo saw noticed that he had a vertical nystagmus that beat downward. A workup revealed that Eduardo had a progressive disease that was damaging the cerebellum, the balance center of the brain. "

BPPV is an unusual medical problem because it can be relieved with simple maneuvers at home. It is also a unique form of vertigo for this reason. Other causes of vertigo do not respond to maneuvers such as the Half Somersault and may need to be treated by a physician. It's important to be able to identify these more serious conditions. This chapter provides guidelines that can help distinguish BPPV from more serious disorders that cause vertigo.

BPPV versus Central Vertigo

The first time a person has an attack of BPPV it's very common to assume that there is something wrong with the brain, such as a tumor, stroke, or multiple sclerosis. However, the vertigo felt during a BPPV attack is actually often more violent than positional vertigo attacks produced by problems in the brain. In addition to the BPPV-induced vertigo being stronger than other forms of vertigo, there are other characteristics that make it possible to tell the difference between BPPV and other forms of vertigo.

The positional vertigo caused by BPPV is much, much more common than positional vertigo that is caused by diseases of the brain, like tumors, strokes, or multiple sclerosis. Most of the time, when people experience a positional vertigo attack, the brain is checked out and found to be normal. The difficult part for patients and their physicians is that vertigo and nystagmus that stems from issues in the brain, which is sometimes referred to as *central vertigo,* is often positional—meaning it can be brought on by position changes, like tilting the head back or lying down flat. The vertigo caused by BPPV is also positional so in this way, central vertigo does mimic BPPV. When vertigo and nystagmus develop for the first time in a person who has not been shown to have BPPV, it's a good idea to have a brain scan such as an MRI or CT scan to ensure there is no tumor, stroke, or other brain disease causing the problem.

Forms of Central Vertigo: Non-BPPV Positional Vertigo and Nystagmus

There are problems in the inner ear that can bring on positional vertigo attacks that are not BPPV and do not result from particles moving in the ear. In this book, we call these kinds of vertigo and the nystagmus that accompanies them *non-BPPV positional nystagmus.* Since vertigo is a feeling, we have to look for physical signs that it is occurring. Recall from Chapter 3, "How Does Vertigo Happen?" that the key physical sign of vertigo is nystagmus (drifting of the eyes). Many researchers like to draw a distinction between BPPV and other forms of positional vertigo by pointing out that BPPV causes a *positioning nystagmus,* which is nystagmus brought on by making a quick head movement. In contrast, non-BPPV sources of vertigo usually cause *positional nystagmus* (which is nystagmus brought on in a certain position of the head, even if the position was reached very slowly).

When people lie down in the dark, if their eye movements are recorded, it is fairly common to see some drifting of the eyes (nystagmus). This drifting may only appear when the person assumes a certain head position, for example, while a person is lying on his or her back with the head turned to the right and not in any other position. In other people, the nystagmus may reverse directions when their heads are turned from side to side or can be present when they are sitting upright as well as when they are lying down. Eye movement observed in people with non-BPPV positional nystagmus lasts much longer than eye movement observed in people with BPPV. Eye movement observed in people with non-BPPV positional nystagmus is also very steady, remaining at the same speed as long as the head is held in one position, or very slowly declines over several minutes.

Eye movement observed in people with non-BPPV positional nystagmus never has the rushed, sudden burst of nystagmus that is seen in people who have BPPV. The movement is also usually horizontal; the eyes drift steadily to the right or to the left, although it can change direction. For example, when a patient is lying down, the eyes may drift rightward when the head is facing right, and leftward when facing left. Often these eye movements are so slow that the person with non-BPPV positional nystagmus is not aware of any feeling of spinning.

Non-BPPV positional nystagmus is very common in people who are recovering from inner ear injuries due to viruses, trauma, or low blood flow. When an injury first occurs, nystagmus is visible when the person has his/her eyes open in the light, and is evident when he/she looks in certain directions. Over the course of a week, the nystagmus will fade in the light, but will still be detectable in recordings in the dark. Often non-BPPV positional nystagmus is stronger when the patient is lying on one side than when they are lying on the other. Over time, non-BPPV positional nystagmus declines until it is only seen when the patient is lying on the worse side. Non-BPPV positional nystagmus can be present many years after the original injury, even though the person may feel fully recovered.

Positional Alcohol-Induced Nystagmus (PAN)

One of the most common forms of non-BPPV positional vertigo is the bed-spinning that people may experience after consuming too much alcohol. This is *Positional Alcohol-Induced Nystagmus*, or

PAN.[1] PAN is primarily due to a small but annoying mechanical problem in the ear.

Ethanol, the type of alcohol in alcoholic beverages, has a lower specific gravity than water. This means that ethanol tends to float in water because it is less dense and lighter in weight than water. When a person drinks, ethanol enters the blood stream, and it makes it way to the inner ears. The sensory organs (ears, eyes, nose, etc.) are well-supplied with blood, so the alcohol quickly enters these organs, including the cupula of the semicircular canal. Under normal circumstances, the cupula has the same density as the endolymph fluid surrounding it and therefore the cupula does not move with gravity. However, when the ethanol enters the ear, the cupula takes up the alcohol quickly—more quickly than the surrounding endolymph fluid. The endolymph fluid is only slowly able to soak up the alcohol from the tissues, so it take hours until the percentage by volume of alcohol in the endolymph fluid and the percentage by volume in the cupula are the same.

This means that the cupula becomes lighter than the fluid that surrounds it and starts to float upward (Figure 5.1 on the next page). As the head is moved from side to side or up and down, the cupula consistently floats up, turning the cupula into a type of gravity sensor. Unfortunately, the semicircular canal only senses spinning and has no ability to sense gravity, so when the cupula floats up, the canal signals a spinning sensation to the brain. This creates the nystagmus of PAN and the awful bed spins. The spins are usually worse when a person lies flat on one side and can be made a bit better by sitting leaning forward with the head propped in the hands.

As time goes by, the amount of ethanol in the endolymph gradually increases so that it begins to equal that in the cupula and in the bloodstream. The spinning becomes less of a problem, and the

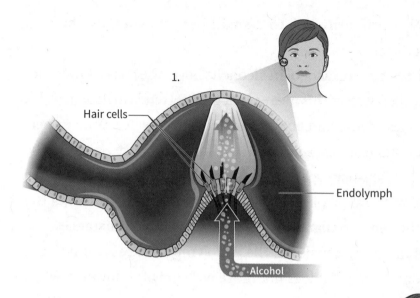

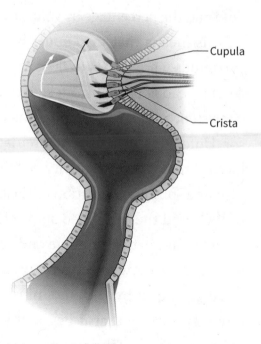

Figure 5.1   Positional Alcohol-Induced Nystagmus. (1) The hair cells of the cupula have excellent blood flow. As a result, alcohol diffuses quickly from the blood to the cupula, but much more slowly to the endolymph surrounding the cupula. The increase in alcohol in the cupula relative to the fluid makes the cupula tend to float in the more-dense endolymph fluid that surrounds the cupula. (2) When a person who has consumed alcohol is lying on one side, the less dense cupula floats up. This movement translates as continuous spinning to the brain and causes vertigo and nystagmus.

person can usually go to sleep. However, a few hours later the level of blood alcohol begins to fall and leaves the cupula quickly through the bloodstream. At this point, there is still plenty of alcohol in the endolymph. This means the cupula is then heavier than the endolymph, and it again becomes a gravity sensor. The spinning returns, often in the early morning hours, giving rise to the classic dizziness of a hangover. One of the popular "cures" for a hangover is "the hair of the dog that bit you." Drinking a Bloody Mary or a shot of alcohol can restore equilibrium between the cupula and the endolymph and alleviate some of the spinning.

The floating cupula mostly causes a horizontal nystagmus in people who suffer from PAN, but all three of the cupulae float, even those in the vertical canals. Alcohol also interferes with eye movement control in the brain; this, combined with floating cupulae, add up to cause the off-balance feeling of drunkenness. Anything that makes the cupula lighter or heavier than the fluid around it can result in positional nystagmus.[2]

Positional Drug-Induced Nystagmus

Dizziness is one of the most frequent side effects of medication. However, even when medications cause dizziness, not many cause nystagmus. So, in most cases, if medication is the root source of dizziness, the room does not appear to spin. That said, there are a few medications that do cause the room to spin; the most common are discussed here. In many instances of *positional drug-induced nystagmus*, nystagmus is present even when the person is sitting or standing, and it is constant, so the symptoms do not resemble BPPV. However, in some of these cases of positional drug-induced nystagmus, nystagmus might be seen when the person is in certain positions; in these instances, the positional drug-induced nystagmus *can* mimic BPPV. This latter kind of positional vertigo does not respond to exercises, however. Lack of response to maneuvers is the tipoff that the problem is not BPPV.

Any drug that is toxic to the ear can cause nystagmus if the drug permanently damages the ear. The most common medications with this adverse effect are *aminoglycoside antibiotics*, particularly *gentamicin*. Usually, when the ear is damaged by this family of medications, a patient experiences dizziness and blurring of vision when the head is moved quickly; but sometimes, especially early in the course of treatment, aminoglycoside antibiotics can also cause nystagmus. Gentamicin is so damaging to the ear that it is even sometimes intentionally injected into injured ears to completely remove balance function (which is called for in some cases). When gentamicin is used in this way, it commonly causes nystagmus.[3] Gentamicin-caused nystagmus is different from BPPV, however, because the gentamicin-caused nystagmus lasts much longer (days or weeks), and nystagmus may be present when the head is upright.

Anticonvulsant medications that are used to treat epileptic seizures can cause nystagmus if patient blood levels become too high. These medications usually cause vertical nystagmus rather than the torsional nystagmus of BPPV.[4] Anticonvulsant-caused nystagmus can be positional and is often worse when the patient is lying down or tipping the head back, but anticonvulsant-caused nystagmus lasts much longer than the brief (30-second) nystagmus that BPPV causes.

Lithium, a medication used to treat bipolar disorder can cause a vertical downbeating nystagmus to develop.[5] This nystagmus may be brought about by head position changes and may be worse when lying down. For this reason, lithium-induced nystagmus can be mistaken for BPPV nystagmus. However, in contrast to BPPV nystagmus, lithium-induced nystagmus is vertical and does not improve with exercises.

Positional Disease-Induced Vertigo and Nystagmus

Sometimes patients or their physicians may mistake a serious brain problem for BPPV. One test for BPPV, the Dix–Hallpike maneuver (see Chapter 2, "The History of BPPV," p. 20), sometimes triggers a form of nystagmus that is caused by a problem, such as a tumor or area of damage in the brain. Usually, this type of nystagmus does not look the same as BPPV nystagmus. However, it can be confusing because the nystagmus of BPPV can vary, depending on which canal is involved, and some forms of BPPV-induced nystagmus are very similar to the nystagmus caused by brain lesions. Brain diseases can also cause positional dizziness without nystagmus. If nystagmus does not occur, brain-related positional dizziness (central vertigo) can be mistaken for mild BPPV.

Multiple sclerosis (MS), a progressive brain disease that can be disabling, can cause a number of abnormal eye movements, including several types of nystagmus.[6] Often, nystagmus is present while the head is upright, not just when lying down. Some of these MS-induced abnormal eye movements can be brought on by simply moving the eyes to the side, up, or down even if the head is held perfectly still. Nystagmus in just one eye can also occur in MS patients but never to people who are suffering from BPPV.

Strokes can result when the brain or brainstem has not received enough blood flow. In these cases, there is a sudden permanent loss of function in that part of the brain.[7] The eye movement and balance pathways travel through the brainstem, so problems with eye movements and balance are some of the most troubling symptoms of strokes. Since stroke damage is permanent, stroke-related vertigo and eye-movement symptoms do not respond to maneuvers and can last months or years. Often eye movement alone will worsen the stroke-related dizziness. Stroke-induced nystagmus can be seen when patients are upright in a seated or standing position.

Degenerative disorders of the brainstem can cause symptoms similar to a stroke, but the symptom tends to come on gradually as the brain deteriorates. Some genetic diseases cause brain cells to die prematurely. These cases begin with a feeling of imbalance that gradually worsens until nystagmus is visible.[8] Often this degeneration results in vertical nystagmus that is present when the head is upright.

Brain tumors can cause symptoms similar to other brain diseases.[9] Depending on how fast a tumor grows, tumor-induced nystagmus can come on suddenly or gradually. Nystagmus in just one eye (similar to the nystagmus that can occur with multiple sclerosis) can be a sign of serious brain problems. As noted earlier in the chapter, when nystagmus develops for the first time in a person who does not obviously have BPPV, it's a good idea to have an MRI or CT scan to ensure there is no brain problem causing the nystagmus and/or vertigo.

Positional Migraine-Induced Vertigo and Nystagmus

Some causes of central vertigo are not harmful to the brain and result in no permanent problems, even though they may feel just as bad as the central vertigo induced by MS or a brain tumor.[10] The most common cause that falls into this category is migraine. (To learn more about migraines and vertigo see Chapter 4, "Non-BPPV Causes of Vertigo," p. 57). People who are experiencing a migraine headache may feel quite dizzy. If these people are examined in darkness with infrared cameras, they sometimes have nystagmus. Migraine-induced vertigo is often more pronounced when lying down, and eye movement can change direction when the headache sufferer rolls from one side to the other. Migraine-induced vertigo and nystagmus are not due to crystals and do not respond to exercises for BPPV. Sleeping until the headache subsides or taking a medicine for motion sickness hastens the resolution of migraine-induced dizziness.

Determining the Difference between BPPV and Central Vertigo

The most important difference between BPPV and central vertigo (which is caused by non-BPPV-related brain problems) is that BPPV can be resolved by doing maneuvers designed to relieve BPPV. Central vertigo caused by brain problems never fully responds to properly performed BPPV maneuvers. A person who feels extremely dizzy and sees the room spinning before BPPV maneuvers and then subsequently feels completely restored after BPPV maneuvers and experiences no more spinning after the maneuvers are complete is very likely to have had BPPV.

That said, some patients think that the BPPV maneuvers helped, but then continue to have some residual dizziness that later turns out to be due to a brain disorder. If you fail to improve after maneuvers, be evaluated by a physician. An evaluation will often include an MRI (magnetic resonance imaging) of the brain. There are differences between BPPV and central vertigo that a trained physician can detect more readily than a lay person. A visit to a physician is always a good idea if BPPV maneuvers do not stop your vertigo.

What are the differences? Central vertigo spells usually last much longer than BPPV episodes. When the room spins with BPPV, it starts slowly, rapidly reaches a peak, and then dies away, all over the course of several seconds. With central vertigo, the perception of spinning continues steadily at the same speed. Central vertigo and nystagmus last for minutes or even remain for as long as the head is kept in the offending position.

In addition, the spinning feels different when it is caused by central vertigo compared to how it feels in BPPV. A person with BPPV usually feels like the room is spinning in a spiral or circle, while central vertigo often makes a patient feel like the room is scrolling straight up or down vertically—almost like a scrolling web page.

There are other difference as well. Central vertigo and nystagmus can be brought on by moving the eyes from side to side or up and down, even if the head is perfectly still. BPPV does not cause an attack unless the head is moved. BPPV also subsides over several seconds if the head is kept still. Moving the eyes can make the nystagmus alter direction slightly during a BPPV attack, but never sets off a new bout of nystagmus. In BPPV of the posterior semicircular canal, looking to the right and left during a bout of nystagmus can change the nystagmus from a circular pattern to a more vertical pattern, but the BPPV nystagmus still dies away after several seconds. And similarly, if BPPV involves the horizontal canal, nystagmus can be changed from right beating to left beating by rolling the head from one side to the other. However, moving only the eyes from right to left and back never causes the nystagmus to change from left beating to right beating in BPPV.

Finally, central vertigo can be triggered by a very slow head movement or a steady head position, while BPPV is set off only by quick movements and goes away even if the head stays in the offending position. To test yourself for central positional vertigo, you can sit upright and very, very slowly move your head until your face is parallel to the ceiling. If the room starts to spin vertically and keeps spinning no matter how long you stay there, it is a sign that the dizziness may be caused by central vertigo. If there is no spinning when you move very slowly, but there is if you move very quickly, then BPPV is more likely the cause.

It is important to recognize that not all positional vertigo is BPPV. Signs that your positional vertigo may be more serious include: dizziness that is set off by very slow head movement changes or by eye movement alone, bouts of spinning that last longer than a few minutes, and nystagmus that is purely vertical. If nystagmus is visible to an observer even when you are upright and not moving, it is not likely to be due to BPPV. The good news is that, most of the time, if lying down makes you dizzy, you probably have BPPV. In the next chapter, we explain why this is so and how crystals tend to get out of place.

6

Why BPPV Happens:
What Did I Do to Get This?

Sheila writes:

> "Yesterday I had to visit the dentist to get a new crown. The work was being done on my upper left back molar so I was reclining in the chair and my head was tilted back. This is never a position I can tolerate for very long. Extreme dizziness and nausea followed the appointment. I found your vertigo maneuver—which I had used successfully in the past—on YouTube. This time I had to perform the maneuver two times, with my husband assisting. I performed it once last night and again this morning. Your Half Somersault is very helpful for me."

If you experience brief spells of spinning when getting out of bed, rolling over, or lying down quickly, it's likely that you have BPPV in the posterior semicircular canal of the ear, and not the more serious central vertigo discussed in Chapter 5, "Central Vertigo: Non-BPPV Positional Vertigo and Nystagmus." (The symptoms of BPPV are reviewed in Chapter 1, "An Introduction to Benign Paroxysmal Positional Vertigo (BPPV).") You are not alone; millions of people suffer from BPPV on any given day. You might wonder why this happened to you. Was it your fault—did you do something to bring this on?

It sometimes seems like physicians, as well as our culture in general, blame patients for their diseases. The media leads us to believe that if we do all the right things, such as exercise, eat the right foods, maintain a healthy weight, and have a good attitude, we'll be completely protected from bad things including heart attacks, cancer, and dementia. People who develop these diseases and other conditions can be seen as failures. Sometimes it seems as if the message is that if only you had worked harder at being healthy, you wouldn't have gotten sick. Sadly, all physicians have seen many, many people who did everything right and still succumbed to a horrendous disease. Many diseases are congenital, or they are caused by injuries, random infections, or other unforeseen events.

The first thing to remember is that, while there are things you can do to prevent BPPV, it is not your fault that you are experiencing BPPV. BPPV can happen when you do perfectly ordinary things that you may have done all your life, and only now do they start to cause problems. The good news is that while BPPV is not your fault, you can make some simple changes that make BPPV less likely to come back. That said, it is pretty difficult to avoid BPPV entirely. It's almost as if BPPV is an occupational hazard of being human.

I've never seen BPPV in an animal except in humans, and this is not just because I am not a veterinarian. Humans are much more likely than other animals to get BPPV because we do things that are outside the "design specs" for our heads. We even sleep in a position that makes the problem worse for us (more on that later in the chapter). We also do some pretty crazy things with our heads, such as doing flips and dangling upside down. This behavior can cause problems for us. We also live longer than most other animals, and BPPV becomes more common with age.

Loose Crystals

The inner ears are filled with a fluid, which is called endolymph, that fills all parts of the inner ear, linking the gravity sensors with the spinning sensors. The fluid also surrounds the otoconia, the little chalk-powder crystals that are supposed to be attached to the gravity sensors, the utricle and saccule. Unfortunately, those otoconia crystals aren't held down by a cargo net; they are just piled in place (Figure 6.1). Stickiness is what usually keeps the crystals where they belong. Each crystal has a thin protein coat that is very gooey, and the

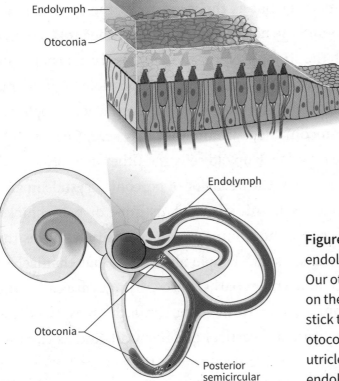

Figure 6.1 Otoconia and endolymph pathways. Our otoconia are piled on the utricle and tend to stick together. However, otoconia can fall off of the utricle and migrate in the endolymph. If otoconia enter a semicircular canal in large enough quantities, BPPV can begin.

membrane the crystals sit on is also very sticky. When experimenters work with these crystals, the otoconia tend to form clumps that stick all over the research instruments and have to be scraped off. Similarly, the crystals stick to each other and to the gravity sensor itself.

It is very difficult to engineer something that stays sticky for years. For example, when you put a Post-it note on the wall next to your desk the first time, it usually stays in place, but as time goes by it gets a lot less sticky. Pretty soon the note will start floating off to the floor when you try to stick it up. The adhesive on the note gradually builds up dust and, at a certain point, the Post-it note simply doesn't stick any longer.

The otoconia crystals are protected from dust because they are enclosed in the inner ear, but as the years go by the otoconia can fracture into pieces and the newly formed edges of the broken pieces are not coated with the sticky protein. The crystals are also not quite as sticky to begin with as, say, Gorilla Glue. It's possible for otoconia crystals to disengage from the gravity sensor even when people are young. When the otoconia float around they may scrape against the walls of the inner ear and pick up old cells and other debris.

Experimenters studying the behavior of otoconia crystals in animals sometimes put small animals, such as mice or baby chicks, into centrifuges, because the spinning of the centrifuge moves the crystals easily off the sensors.[1] People also like to put themselves into centrifuges. At amusement parks, the centrifuges are called the Round Up, Zero Gravity, the Tornado, or similar names. On these rides, people stand against a vertical circular wall, and as the ride spins and the floor of the ride drops away, the carnival attendees are pinned against the wall by centrifugal force. As it spins, a ride like this creates the illusion that riders are lying on their backs, even though they start out upright. This is because rides like this shift the otoconia crystals on the inner ear's gravity sensors so effectively. No one has ever been able to look inside the ear to see how many crystals fall off the sensors when a person rides this sort of ride, but it doesn't take much movement and force to remove crystals. Just hitting your head can remove crystals.[2] People who hit their heads hard in a car accident can loosen their crystals and slipping and falling in the bathroom can be enough to detach otoconia crystals. If you crawl under your desk to find a dropped pen and you bump your head on the desk when you try to stand up, the resulting jar is probably enough to remove crystals. This means that sooner or later, most people have some crystals floating loose that are no longer stuck to the gravity sensors. And because the endolymph fluid pathways travel throughout the inner ear, these loose crystals have a liquid path to just about anywhere.

Of course, animals slip and fall too, and can hit their heads. Imagine the forces that impact the crystals in the head of a bighorn sheep during rutting season. The rams butt heads hard enough to hear the crack a mile away. Why don't these animals fall down constantly as they battle vertigo? As you will see in the rest of this chapter, there is a little more to the story than simply loose crystals.

Head Position

It takes more than loose crystals to trigger BPPV. To be at risk for BPPV, you must have loose crystals *and* you must position your head in just the right way to move those loose crystals into one of your spinning sensors. The ears of animals—especially the ears of other mammals—are not built that differently from ours. If other animals had been getting BPPV for millions of years, there probably would have been some evolutionary pressure to correct the design flaw that allows loose crystals to enter the semicircular canal in human ears. Since other animals don't experience BPPV, and since BPPV isn't fatal, there isn't much evolutionary pressure to change the human inner ear structure. Humans, like many animals, have a built-in design flaw. If we all have this flaw, how do animals avoid getting BPPV?

Other mammals do not make the sort of head movements that humans do. Think about your last trip to the zoo. You probably saw some animals sleeping. What position are animals' heads in when they sleep? Many sleep standing up. Some lie with their heads on their paws, or they lie on their side. How many animals have you seen lying flat on their back, with their nose pointing in the sky? I've seen some primates in this position, but I've never seen an elephant, zebra, or antelope sleep the way humans do. Yet we humans absolutely love this position. Every night, year after year, people lie flat on their backs looking up at the ceiling. We roll from side to side during the night, tossing and turning. Each time we roll over, the otoconia crystals shift in our inner ears. This would not be a problem if not for a little design flaw in every mammal's ears (Figure 6.2).

The inner ear senses spinning when endolymph fluid moves within the semicircular canals. The canals are rings that contain the spinning sensors. The rings are not complete circles; about one quarter of each ring is open to the cavity that contains the gravity sensors with their attached crystals. Unfortunately for humans, these openings lie just above and behind the gravity sensors in the skull. This means when we lie flat on our backs, the openings are below the level of the sensors. Because the crystals are relatively heavy, gravity can pull any detached crystals down into the semicircular canals when a person is lying down. Tossing and turning helps stir up any loose crystals, so our nighttime restlessness increases the likelihood of a problem.

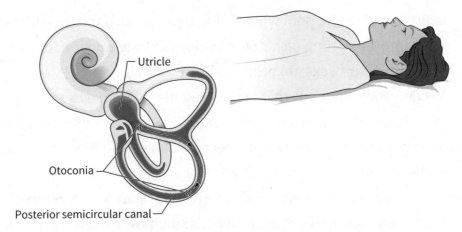

Figure 6.2   The relationship between the utricle and the semicircular canals. When a person is lying flat on the back facing the ceiling, the otoconia can fall into the opening to the semicircular canals.

Crystals can fall into the canals any time the head is horizontal to the floor, such as when the head is tipped back so the nose is facing straight up, parallel to the ceiling. Moving your head past the horizontal when you are on your back, so that your chin is pointing toward the ceiling, worsens the problem. Dangling your head upside down, either forward or back, also moves the crystals to a position just above the openings to the canals. People who don't have any loose otoconia crystals can safely do flips and dangle their heads, but once the crystals become loose, these movements can cause BPPV.

Some people have occupations that require them to move their heads in a way that moves crystals easily. These people get BPPV more than other people their age who don't move their heads in this way. For example, drill sergeants and exercise trainers that regularly do multiple vigorous sit-ups or toe-touches are susceptible to BPPV. Yoga instructors put their heads upside down frequently and this makes them more likely to have BPPV as well. Swimmers who do flips at the end of the pool while doing laps can also move otoconia crystals into the wrong place. Mechanics working under cars while lying flat on their backs are prone to BPPV as well.

When people find out that something like yoga makes you more likely to have BPPV, they often become upset. Yoga is supposed to be good for you! It's exercise! But just because something is good for one part of your body doesn't mean it's great for every part. Running is great for your heart but not necessarily as great for your knees. Similarly, yoga and other exercises that involve striking poses where your head is lying flat on the ground or upside down are not great for your inner ears. Inner ears work best when they are located in upright heads.

Just like work positions or poses, everyday actions can also move crystals. Many people like to flip their heads upside down while blowing their hair dry. This is a great way to move loose crystals into canals. When you are connecting cords or cables under your desk or working on pipes under the sink, you may tip your head from side to side while your head is down or horizontal. That movement can shift your otoconia crystals. Even going to the hair salon can dislodge crystals. A stylist may tip your head back into the sink and jiggle it back and forth as they wash your hair and scrub your scalp. This movement can be enough to move particles.

Sometimes the crystals are moved by things you can't avoid. Dentists often tip patients back so the head is down and turned to one side and then place vibrating objects such as dental drills against the jaw. (This is what happened to Shiela in the chapter-opening story.) This is a perfect way to move particles into the canals. During surgery, the head is often placed flat and even tipped backward without a pillow, and may be held in this position for hours. It's not uncommon for surgical patients to wake up with BPPV after surgery for this reason.

Brain surgery is especially likely to result in BPPV both because of the head position and the application of vibrating drills against the skull.

Once the crystals enter the semicircular canals, you are set up to have an attack of BPPV. Of course, it takes a large clump of crystals to cause enough vertigo that your eyes spin and you see the room spin along with them. You might have just a few crystals in your canals without knowing it, and it will only be after more have joined them that you will have your first attack.

Most people don't experience BPPV until they are older, and even then, not everyone gets it.[3] It isn't practical to restrict head movements and positions to try to prevent BPPV. Even after you suffer your first attack of BPPV, indicating that you have loose crystals, it's unrealistic to try to stop making all the movements that displace particles. However, when practical, you should make the effort to restrict any of these movements that are easy to avoid. In Chapter 12, "Troubleshooting," we offer practical advice to reduce the risk of recurrences.

Remember that it is not your fault you have BPPV. It's a design flaw in your head that you share with all humans and many animals, too. A number of random, minor things act together to cause BPPV.

Now that you know more about why people experience BPPV, we move on to resolving the problem. The Half Somersault maneuver removes particles from the posterior canal, which is the semicircular canal most likely to be the culprit when BPPV strikes. Although BPPV most often stems from problems in the posterior canal, we all have six canals in our heads (three in each ear) and otoconia crystals can find their way into any of the six or in more than one of them. Different maneuvers are needed to move crystals found in each of the canals. Reading the next chapter will help you locate the problem crystals in your ear.

7

The Half Somersault Maneuver

Eliza writes:

"On December 24th, I woke up with my room ferociously spinning around me. I crawled to the bathroom unable to keep food or fluids in my system. I was clueless about what was going on, I was scared and miserable. I had experienced briefer, less powerful bouts of dizziness and nausea three or four times before but nothing like this. I thought this was my last day on earth! On top of everything, this was Christmas Eve. I ended up in an ER wishing Merry Christmas to the emergency staff. The worst part was that I couldn't care less that it was Christmas—I just wanted to feel better. The doctor, who was really good, I thought, diagnosed me with vertigo (something I'd never heard before), gave me valium, and sent me home when I felt better with a prescription of diazepam. She told me to take it if the symptoms persist. I did not like the diazepam part! I'm not big on taking medications.

The next day I woke up and, thank God, the nausea had disappeared but I was still staggering around the house like a drunk sailor. My symptoms kind of matched the description of BPPV I found online and I went on an internet hunt for treatment. Your article, 'An Easy Fix for Vertigo,' was the first title that caught my attention. The fact that you specialize in something that you actually suffered from yourself gave me a huge hope. The movement that you came up with and your explanation seemed so simple and understandable that I was determined: I decided to put an end to my problem once and for all! The worst thing I thought that might happen was that I might throw up again—not a big deal at this point.

I lifted my head up. The sensation that you describe was there! This was already working. Yay! I put my head down and the end of the world came! The spinning was so unbearable that I said to myself, "Wonderful! This is the position that I'm going to be in as I take my last breath!" I stayed like that with my butt up and my teeth clenched waiting to see if I would come out of the maneuver alive.

I did come out alive and with the most unimaginable relief! I slept the way you suggested (my left ear was the affected one. I figured that out also, thanks to you). I did the exercise four times and now I feel like a brand-new person!**"**

The Half Somersault maneuver arose out of a very practical problem I encountered in my professional practice as a neurotologist and practicing physician. The problem I needed to solve was straightforward: I was seeking a way for people with BPPV to resolve their vertigo without having to wait to see a provider. I knew from my own experience that when you are struck by BPPV, you need help instantly. It's just too horrible to have to make an appointment that might be days or weeks later, or to drag yourself in to a clinic when you're already suffering enough. Once I learned how to do the Half Somersault maneuver on myself, and then did a research study that proved my maneuver worked, I was ready to share it with all the people dealing with BPPV. [1]

When you wake up with vertigo, you want to be free of the symptoms as quickly as possible. In theory, the perfect maneuver is one that is quick and easy to do alone, has a high rate of success, causes no dizziness, and has no risk of complications. This is a tall order. Any time the particles in the inner ear move, a person with BPPV will experience at least some dizziness. In addition, when particles move in the ear, they can easily leave one place and enter another location that is even worse. It's also hard to remember how to do any movement by yourself while you are experiencing severe vertigo. It is especially difficult getting your head into a specific, exact position without anyone to help you. All of these issues must be addressed and weighed in the search for the best possible solution to the problem.

The Advantages of the Half Somersault Maneuver

The Half Somersault maneuver is designed to allow people to remove particles from the semicircular canals by themselves, without anyone else present to help. It is also designed to help prevent particles from falling into the horizontal canal after they have been removed from the posterior canal. Recall from Chapter 1, "An Introduction to Benign Paroxysmal Positional Vertigo (BPPV)," that this is the major complication of other maneuvers. (I discuss this complication in more detail in Chapter 9, "Unusual Forms of BPPV".) I devised the Half Somersault as an alternative to the other established maneuvers in an effort to specifically avoid that complication and therefore to create a maneuver that is safer to perform. The way the Half Somersault maneuver is carried out is also specifically designed to help the sufferer experience less severe vertigo during the maneuver than he or she would feel when doing the other common maneuvers. For this reason, the Half Somersault maneuver is easier to tolerate, and yet it still succeeds in moving the particles out of the posterior canal.[2]

Determining Which Ear Is Your Problem Ear

Before beginning to perform the Half Somersault maneuver, you need to have some idea which ear has the loose crystals present and is therefore the problem ear. In general, if you feel most dizzy when lying down with your head turned to the right, the problem is probably in your right ear. If you feel worse when lying on your left side, then it's probably in your left ear.

If you cannot tell from just lying on both sides or are not sure, try the Dix–Hallpike maneuver (see Chapter 2, "The History of BPPV," p. 20: Sit on the edge of your bed, turn your head toward your right shoulder, and fall back onto the bed, keeping your head turned to the right. If this causes the room to spin, you have BPPV in the right ear. If not, repeat the same moves with your head turned to the left. If this causes the room to spin, you have BPPV in the left ear.

It is possible to have BPPV in both ears, but most people typically only have one affected ear. If you can't tell which ear has particles in the canal, you can still treat the problem. Start by treating the right ear and if you still feel badly after that treatment, repeat the maneuver for the left ear. Keep alternating until all your symptoms are gone.

Performing the Half Somersault Maneuver: Step-by-Step

Step 1. The first step in the Half Somersault is to kneel on your hands and knees on the floor. You can also get on your hands and knees in the middle of a large bed if you have bad knees or trouble getting up and down off the floor. Put a trash can near you if you are sensitive to dizziness; you may get nauseated or even vomit when doing maneuvers. You are going to experience dizziness, but this is a good thing because it indicates that the particles are moving toward the canal exit and back to where they belong.

Step 2. You are now in the proper position to begin moving the particles out of your canal. While you are still in the kneeling position, quickly tip your head up until your eyes are looking straight up at the ceiling (Figure 7.1). It is OK to rock back to kneel on your heels to get your head positioned far enough back to see the ceiling. Your head should be centered, not turned to either side. After tipping your head back, you might experience a couple of seconds of dizziness. It's OK to close

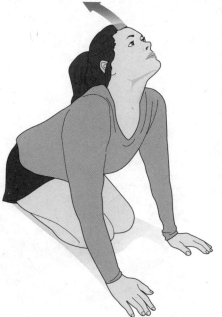

Figure 7.1 The Half Somersault: Steps 1 and 2. Get on your hands and knees on the floor. Rock back into a kneeling position and quickly tilt your head and look up at the ceiling, tipping your head back as far as possible.

your eyes, but don't move or lower your head—just keep it tilted up. This position helps dislodge the particles and gets them moving. Moving quickly helps to get the crystals in motion. Stay in this position for 30 seconds, or until all the spinning has stopped.

Step 3. Without turning your head to either side, lean forward and get on your hands and knees as if you are about to do a somersault. Place your head completely upside down in front of your knees, supporting yourself with both hands on either side of your head (Figure 7.2). You don't have to move quickly during this step, taking a few seconds to get into this position is just fine. Once your head is upside down, you may feel more spinning. It may be very intense or it may be milder than your previous spells. Hold this position and wait for the spinning to slow down. Stay in this position for at least 30 seconds, or as long as you must in order for the spinning to stop.

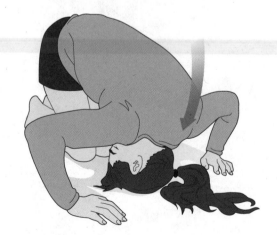

Figure 7.2   The Half Somersault: Step 3. On all fours, get in a position as if you were about to do a somersault. Your hands and knees will support you when the spinning begins. You may feel vertigo that will last up to 30 seconds.

Step 4. The next step is to prepare to flush the particles out of the canal. You'll need to line up your canals so that when your head is lifted, the movement of the fluid in the canal flushes all the particles out. To do this, turn your head so that you are looking at the elbow that is on the same side of your body as the problem ear. If the problem is with your right ear, look at the right elbow (Figure 7.3). If your problem is in the left ear, look at your left elbow. (If you are not certain, first treat the right side and then treat the left side if you still are experiencing symptoms.) Turn far enough so your head is turned about half way to your shoulder. Stay in this position long enough to make sure all the spinning has subsided completely before doing the next movement.

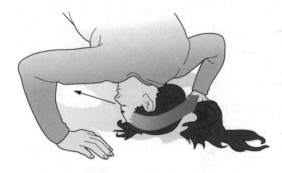

Figure 7.3   The Half Somersault: Step 4. Note that these figures illustrate treatment of the right ear. If you think you have BPPV in the right ear, while your head is upside down, turn to face your right elbow. Your head should be turned about halfway to your right shoulder. If you have BPPV in the left ear, turn to face your left ear (see Figure 7.6 on p. 99).

Step 5. The next "flushing-out" steps should be done quickly. The fluid must move in a wave in order for the particles to start moving and keep moving out of the canal. Keeping your head turned to face your elbow, quickly lift your head until it is level with

Figure 7.4 The Half Somersault: Step 5. Note that these figures illustrate treatment of the right ear. While still in the upside-down position, keeping the head turned toward the right elbow, quickly lift your head until it is level with your back. Your head should be level with your back and still be turned toward the right elbow when you are done.

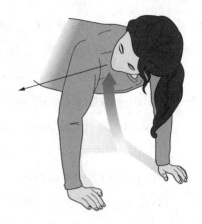

your back (Figure 7.4). You might feel a rush of dizziness as you do this. If this happens, don't alter your position. Keep your head turned toward your elbow and level with your back and wait for the dizziness to subside. Stay in this position for about 30 seconds, until the spinning has stopped.

Step 6. The final step is to return your head to the upright position and your body to a kneeling position. Keeping your head turned to the side, quickly lift your head fully upright, pushing yourself up with your hands so you end up kneeling (Figure 7.5). Another wave of dizziness might occur. Wait until all your dizziness ends before changing your head position again.

Figure 7.5 The Half Somersault: Step 6. Note that these figures illustrate treatment of the right ear. Still looking at your right elbow, rock back onto your knees to bring your head fully upright while keeping it turned to the right. This step should be performed quickly.

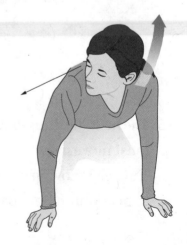

Step 7. After the maneuver is complete, remain in a kneeling position and wait to determine if all your dizziness has passed. Move your head from side to side or up and down: Do you feel normal now, or is there still some spinning? If you can't trigger any spinning and you feel better, you don't need to repeat the maneuver. However, most people have to do the maneuver more than once—on average about four times—in order to get every last particle out. After a couple of minutes, if you still feel dizzy and you think there are still particles in the ear, repeat the maneuver. If you have BPPV in the left ear, follow the instructions for the maneuver shown in Figure 7.6.

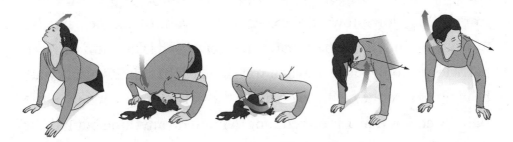

Figure 7.6   The Half Somersault. This sequence illustrates how to treat the left ear. The key change is that you face the left elbow when upside down, and the head remains turned toward the left elbow throughout the rest of the exercise.

You can see all the steps of the Half Somersault Maneuver on pages 106–107 (right ear) and 108–109 (left ear).

An Internal View of the Half Somersault Maneuver

It is informative and helpful to know what is happening during each step of the Half Somersault maneuver and how the maneuver is working to address your problem. At the start of the maneuver, when your head is upright and you are kneeling, the loose particles are located in the lowest part of the ear: the posterior semicircular canal, at a spot just beyond the sensor. In order to get them out, you have to move them all around the loop of the canal, a journey that is more than 180 degrees.

Tipping your head up in Step 2 starts the particles moving. This move has to be done quickly because the particles are sticky and can stay attached to the lining of the canal unless they are jostled loose with a jerking movement. The particles are in a circular tube that curves upward at the bottom. Imagine turning this tube upside down. The particles would then be balanced on top of a curved hill and could roll either out (which you want) or down the other side back toward the sensor (which you don't want). To prevent them from rolling down toward the sensor, you want to get the particles moving around the loop so that, when your head is upside down, the particles can only move the right way: toward the exit. By tilting your head up to face the ceiling, you move the particles far enough in the right direction that it is difficult for them to do anything but fall out during the next step (Figure 7.7).

When you put your head upside down in Step 3, the particles should be far enough around the curve of the canal that their only option is to fall down toward the exit (Figure 7.8). Gravity should do all the work, but it has to contend with the fluid in your ears. As you put your head upside down, the fluid is moving against the particles as they start to fall. This slows them down a little, and since the speed of the spinning sensation is related to how quickly the particles move, this can decrease the intensity of the vertigo you feel. Once your head is fully upside down and not moving any longer, the particles pick up speed as gravity continues to pull them down in the canal. After several seconds, they reach the new lowest part of the

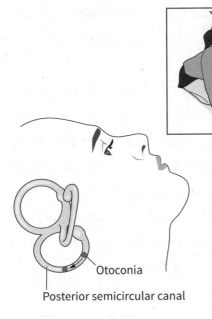

Figure 7.7 Half Somersault internal view: Steps 1 and 2. When the head is tipped back, the crystals start moving toward the exit of the canal. Keeping the head tipped up allows the otoconia to move to the part of the canal that is lowest when your head is tipped. This moves the crystals about one quarter of the distance they need to travel to make it to the exit.

Otoconia

Posterior semicircular canal

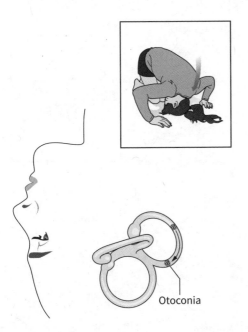

Figure 7.8 The Half Somersault internal view: Step 3. When your head is upside-down, the crystals fall to the new lowest part of the canal, which is now very near the exit. This moves the crystals about three quarters of the distance they need to travel to make it to the exit. During this time, you will experience some vertigo. As you move your head into the upside-down position, the fluid in your ears slows the movement of the falling crystals.

Otoconia

canal. (This new lowest part of the canal is really the top, near the exit, when your head is right-side up.) The spinning wanes and stops once the particles stop moving.

By turning your head to face your elbow in Step 4, you are lining the canal up so that it is in the exact plane of movement when you next raise your head (Figure 7.9). The *sagittal plane* is the plane running down the middle of your head and body. It is the imaginary plane that divides your body into two halves right between your eyes, through your nose, lips, and chin and down through your belly button. The posterior canal that you are trying to empty out is in a plane lying at 45 degrees to this sagittal plane. To flush something out of your right posterior canal, for example, you have to turn your head 45 degrees to the right to line up the right posterior canal so that it is parallel to this plane. By turning your head until you are looking at your elbow, you are turning your head about 45 degrees, so it is correctly positioned for the next step.

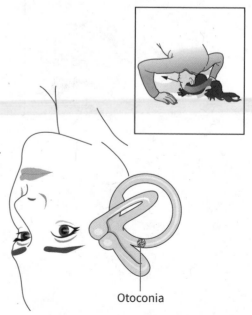

Figure 7.9   The Half Somersault internal view: Step 4. Note that these figures illustrate treatment of the right ear. When your head is turned to the right, all up-and-down head movements move fluid in the right posterior semicircular canal. This helps dislodge crystals in the posterior canal of the right ear and allows them to fall out easily. (See Figure 7.6 on p. 103 for treatment of the left ear.)

Otoconia

Quickly moving your head to shoulder level from the upside-down position in Step 5 moves your head in the sagittal plane. Since the canal is now lined up with this plane (because your head is turned to face your elbow), this movement causes the fluid to move in the canal in the direction of the exit. By moving quickly, you push this fluid outward against the particles, flushing the particles toward the exit (Figure 7.10). Sometimes the particles depart the canal entirely during this step, but they have a long way to travel—almost a full circle before they reach the exit—so you still want to complete the entire maneuver.

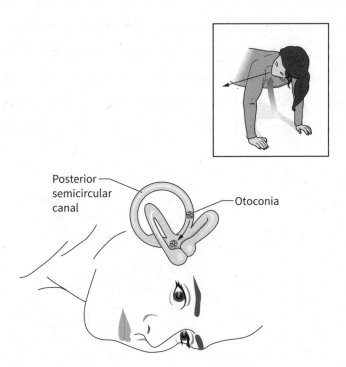

Posterior semicircular canal

Otoconia

Figure 7.10   The Half Somersault internal view: Step 5. When you quickly raise your head to shoulder level, this flushes the fluid and crystals in the posterior canal almost the remainder of the distance around the curved canal toward the exit. At the end of this step, the crystals will be almost all of the way out of the canal.

As long as your head remains turned, your canal is still in the sagittal plane and the canal is further flushed out when you lift your head. As you again lift your head from shoulder level to a fully upright position in Step 6, the fluid again flushes toward the exit of the canal, and any remaining particles are flushed out with it (Figure 7.11). This can cause brief dizziness during this step. Sometimes the spinning will suddenly stop just after you become upright. This may indicate that all the particles have exited the canal and that you do not need to do another maneuver.

Many people ask why they have to repeat this maneuver. Why don't all the particles get flushed out the first time? Sometimes they do. However, keep in mind that there may be many particles, possibly even hundreds, forming one or several clumps. And it is impossible to know how many particles there are and exactly where they are located in the canal. You can't look inside your head to see how many clumps there are or if you've got everything lined up perfectly as you complete the maneuver.

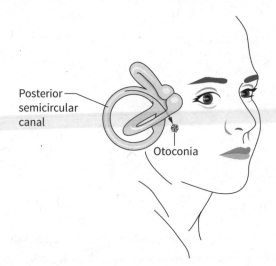

Posterior semicircular canal

Otoconia

Figure 7.11 The Half Somersault internal view: Step 6. Quickly raising your head while it is turned to the right flushes the fluid and crystals out of the exit to the right canal and prevents the crystals from falling back into the canal.

It is easier to get one clump out than to flush out 10 clumps. The more particles and clumps that you have, the stronger the vertigo will be, so if you experience strong spinning during one pass through the maneuver, it often means that you are making a lot of progress during that pass and you will experience a lot of relief once it is done. In addition, some particles may stick along the edge of the canal until you've shaken them loose with a few maneuvers. Because the canal is so curved, some fall back in toward the sensor instead of moving toward the exit when you put your head upside down. If everything isn't aligned perfectly, particles can move the wrong way, or not move at all.

After a successful maneuver, you will feel less spinning in subsequent passes through the maneuver. In this way, the maneuver "rewards" you for a good job. It's best to do several maneuvers in a row to get everything cleared out all at once. However, the spinning also sets off nausea, so you may need to stop if you get too queasy. You can always do another set the next day or take a medicine to reduce nausea and repeat the exercise an hour later if your dizziness has not resolved.

This chapter covered the basics about how to perform the Half Somersault maneuver. You can also find several videos of the Half Somersault maneuver on various online sites including YouTube (https://tinyurl.com/kqa8u5s). These videos show people actually doing the maneuver.

It is important to note that not everyone with BPPV can tolerate the positions included in the maneuver. People with bad knees and bad backs have trouble getting on their hands and knees, even though they are just as likely to get BPPV as anyone else. To help these people, I have created some variations of the Half Somersault that allow people with movement issues to find relief. These are covered in the next chapter.

Half Somersault Maneuver: Right Ear

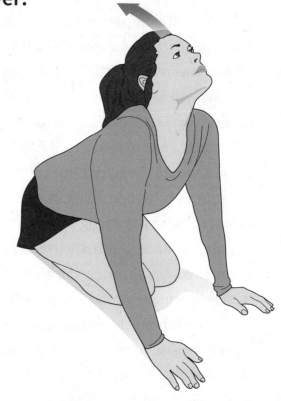

Steps 1 and 2. Get on your hands and knees on the floor. Rock back into a kneeling position and quickly tilt your head and look up at the ceiling, tipping your head back as far as possible.

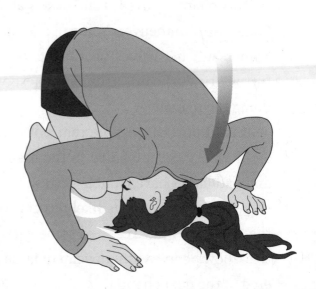

Step 3. On all fours, get in a position as if you were about to do a somersault. Your hands and knees will support you when the spinning begins. You may feel vertigo that will last up to 30 seconds.

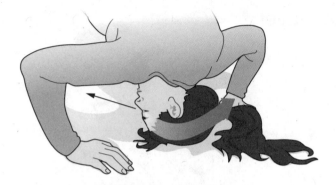

Step 4. While your head is upside down, turn to face your right elbow. Your head should be turned about halfway to your right shoulder.

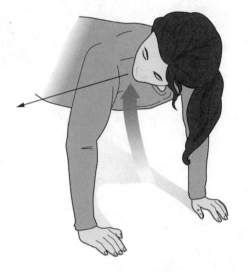

Step 5. While still in the upside-down position, keeping the head turned toward the right elbow, quickly lift your head until it is level with your back. Your head should be level with your back and still be turned toward the right elbow when you are done.

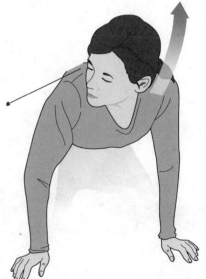

Step 6. Still looking at your right elbow, rock back onto your knees to bring your head fully upright while keeping it turned to the right. This step should be performed quickly.

Half Somersault Maneuver: Left Ear

Steps 1 and 2. Get on your hands and knees on the floor. Rock back into a kneeling position and quickly tilt your head and look up at the ceiling, tipping your head back as far as possible.

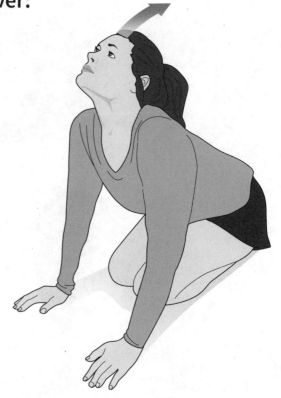

Step 3. On all fours, get in a position as if you were about to do a somersault. Your hands and knees will support you when the spinning begins. You may feel vertigo that will last up to 30 seconds.

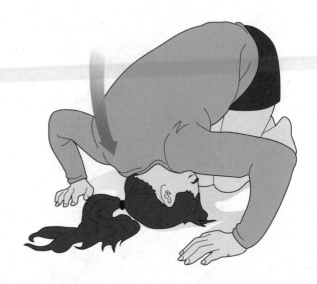

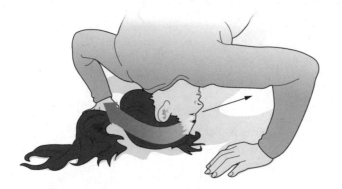

Step 4. While your head is upside down, turn to face your left elbow. Your head should be turned about halfway to your left shoulder.

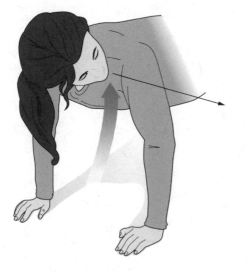

Step 5. While still in the upside-down position, keeping the head turned toward the left elbow, quickly lift your head until it is level with your back. Your head should be level with your back and still be turned toward the left elbow when you are done.

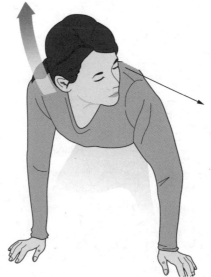

Step 6. Still looking at your left elbow, rock back onto your knees to bring your head fully upright while keeping it turned to the left. This step should be performed quickly.

8

Variations of the Half Somersault Maneuver

> " Nicholas, a man in his seventies, came in to BPPV clinic with a story of experiencing very typical brief spells of vertigo when he lay down with his right ear on the pillow. He had seen the Half Somersault maneuver video online, but he had been afraid to try the exercise because he had very bad knees. It was too painful for him to kneel on the floor and it was hard for him to get back up from the floor. I was able to resolve his vertigo with maneuvers in the clinic, but he needed an at-home exercise that spared his knees. After we taught Nicholas a seated variation of the Half Somersault maneuver, he was able to do exercises whenever he needed them at home. "

After reading Chapter 7, "The Half Somersault Maneuver," you now know how to do the Half Somersault maneuver, but if you think it's too difficult to get in the positions described in that chapter, you will need this chapter. In this chapter, we present and describe versions of the Half Somersault for less-mobile people.

Not everyone is flexible enough to fold themselves into a pretzel, and for people with stiff or painful joints—especially if those joints are in the back or neck—it can be hard to tolerate BPPV maneuvers.

Since flexibility limitations tend to come on with age, just like BPPV, it means the very people who need maneuvers most are often the ones that have trouble tolerating them. Thankfully, although the Half Somersault maneuver requires that people put their bodies in certain positions, it is really only the head movements that matter when it comes to treating BPPV. The head movements are what cause the particles to rotate; the body positions only exist to make it simple and easy to achieve these head positions. Fortunately, there are other ways to achieve these same head movements and positions. Before performing any of these maneuvers, follow the procedure in Chapter 7, "The Half Somersault Maneuver," starting on p. 98 to determine which side your problem is on.

Seated Half Somersault Maneuver

If you cannot get on your knees because they are stiff or sore, or you have trouble getting up from the floor, the Half Somersault maneuver can be done on a bed so that your knees are cushioned. If even this results in too much pain, you can try doing the modified, seated Half Somersault maneuver presented here while seated in a chair. You will need to know which ear is affected because you will turn your head to that side during the maneuver (to the right if it is the right ear, to the left if it is the left ear). If you review Chapter 7, "The Half Somersault Maneuver," and are still unsure which ear has loose crystals, perform the maneuver once to the right, then again to the left.

To perform the seated Half Somersault maneuver, place a sturdy chair alongside a bed or sofa so you can rest your hand on it to steady yourself. Then complete the following steps:

Step 1. Sit normally with knees apart, facing forward in the chair. Rest your elbow on the sofa or on the bed next to you.

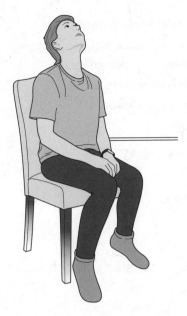

Figure 8.1   Seated Half Somersault: Steps 1 and 2. Tip your head up and as far back as possible. Some spinning sensations may occur in this position.

Step 2. Quickly tip your head straight up so your eyes are looking directly at the ceiling (Figure 8.1). Your head should be centered, not turned to either side. After doing this, you might experience a couple of seconds of dizziness. It's OK to close your eyes but don't lower your head or move—keep your head tilted up. Wait in this position for at least 30 seconds, or until all the spinning stops.

Step 3. Next, without turning your head to either side, lean forward in the chair and bend at the waist until your head is nearly upside down between your knees (Figure 8.2 on the next page). Keep one hand on the arms of the chair or the bed to steady yourself. Once your head is upside down, you may feel spinning. Wait in this position for the spinning to slow down. You'll need to stay in this position for at least 30 seconds.

Figure 8.2   Seated Half Somersault: Step 3. Bend forward and place your head upside down between your knees. A spinning sensation is likely to occur in this position. The spinning should last less than 30 seconds.

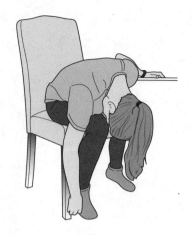

Once the spinning stops, reach down with both hands to touch your toes.

Step 4. The next step is preparing to flush the particles out of the canal. You must line up your canals so that when your head is lifted, the fluid movement will flush the particles out. To do this, hang your arms down toward the floor and turn your head so that you are looking at the inside of your elbow on the same side of your body as the problem ear (Figure 8.3). If your problem is in your right ear, look at your right elbow. If

Figure 8.3   Seated Half Somersault: Step 4. Let your arms dangle down to touch the floor. Turn your head to look at your right elbow if you are treating the right ear.

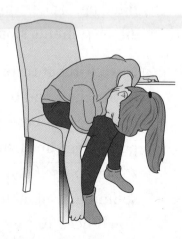

your problem is in your left ear, look at your left elbow. (If you are not certain, treat the right side during the first maneuver and then treat the left side with a second maneuver if you still have any symptoms.) Remain with your head in this in the upside-down position until all the spinning has completely subsided before going on to the next step.

Step 5. These next flushing-out steps should be completed quickly. Keeping your head turned to face your elbow, quickly lift your head so it is level with your back and your head is horizontal (Figure 8.4). You might experience a rush of dizziness as you do this. If this happens, keep your head turned toward your elbow and wait for the dizziness to subside. Stay in this position for about 30 seconds, until any spinning has stopped. You may feel more secure resting your hand on the bed or sofa once you have reached this position.

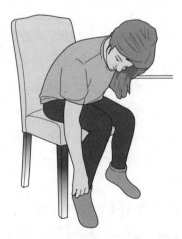

Figure 8.4   Seated Half Somersault: Step 5. Lift your head so that it is in a straight line with your back, horizontal to the floor. The head should remain turned to the right if your right ear is being treated.

Figure 8.5   Seated Half Somersault:
Step 6. Lift your head and sit fully
upright, keeping the head turned to the
right. Wait for any dizziness to cease
and then face forward. The maneuver
is completed at this point.

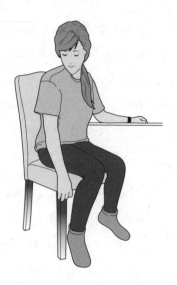

Step 6. The final step is to return to the upright position (Figure 8.5).
Keeping your head turned to the side, quickly lift your head
fully upright, so you are sitting upright in the chair with your
head turned to the side. Another wave of dizziness might
occur. Wait until any dizziness subsides before turning your
head to face forward.

After completing all the steps of the maneuver, tip your head up
and down a few times. If you don't feel dizzy any longer, you may not
need to do another maneuver. If you still experience a spinning sensation when you move your head, repeat the steps of the maneuver.
Most people have to repeat the maneuver a few times to flush out all
the particles.

Standing Half Somersault Maneuver

If you have trouble bending your knees at all but still have a flexible
neck and back, a variation of the Half Somersault maneuver can be
done while standing. However, it is important to note that standing

during the maneuver leaves you more vulnerable to falling. To be safe, perform the maneuver near a low bed, a padded armchair, or a recliner, and, if possible, have someone with you to act as a spotter. Facing the side of your bed or the seat of the recliner is best, because if you fall from this position, the bed or chair will be there to support you. Patients have informed me that they have performed the Half Somersault maneuver at a gym leaning over an exercise bar at hip height. If you try this, be sure there is a mat under you in case you fall and have someone with you to act as a spotter.

To perform the standing Half Somersault maneuver, complete the following steps.

Step 1. Stand facing a bed or chair. Place one hand on the surface in front of you to steady yourself. Quickly tip your head up so your eyes are looking directly at the ceiling (Figure 8.6). You should be facing straight up with your head centered, not turned to either side. You might experience a few seconds of dizziness. It's OK to close your eyes if you have a

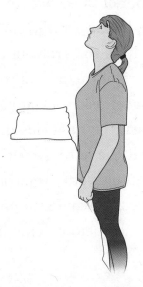

Figure 8.6 Standing Half Somersault: Step 1. Tip your head up and back as far as possible. This may cause a brief spell of spinning. The spinning indicates the particles have begun moving toward the exit.

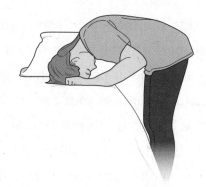

Figure 8.7 Standing Half Somersault: Step 2. Place your head upside down touching the bed or chair seat. Hold your hands on either side of your head to steady yourself.

spotter to hold on to but don't lower your head or move— keep your head tilted straight up. Hold this position for 30 seconds, or until all the spinning has stopped.

Step 2. In Step 2, without turning your head to either side, lean forward and bend over until your head is nearly upside down on the bed or chair seat. Put both your hands on either side of your head to steady yourself (Figure 8.7). Once your head is upside down, you may feel the spinning sensation. Hold this position for at least 30 seconds or until the spinning slows and ceases.

Step 3. Next, prepare to flush the particles out of the canal. To do this, turn your head so that you are looking at the elbow that is on the same side of your body as the problem ear (Figure 8.8). If the problem is in your right ear, look at your right elbow. If the problem is in your left ear, look at your left elbow. (If you are not certain, treat the right side during the first maneuver and then treat the left side with a second maneuver if you have any symptoms after you complete the first maneuver.) Hold this position and wait until all the spinning has completely subsided before doing the next movement.

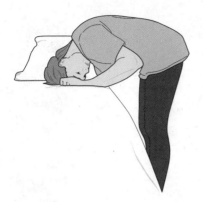

Figure 8.8   Standing Half Somersault: Step 3. Turn your head to the right if you are treating your right ear and to the left if you are treating the left ear. Look directly at the inside of your elbow.

Step 4. These flushing-out steps should be executed quickly. Keeping your head turned to face the elbow on the side with the problem, quickly lift your head so it is level with your back (Figure 8.9) and in a straight line with your spine. You might experience a rush of dizziness as you do this. Try to ignore the dizziness and hold your head at back level turned toward your elbow. Hold this position for at least 30 seconds, until any spinning stops. Keep your hands on the bed or chair seat to support yourself.

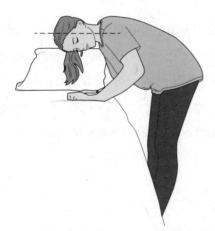

Figure 8.9   Standing Half Somersault: Step 4. Quickly lift your head until it is in a straight line with your spine. Keep your head turned to the side you are treating (left in this picture).

Figure 8.10   Standing Half Somersault: Step 5. Stand up quickly keeping your head turned to the side you are treating (the left side in this example).

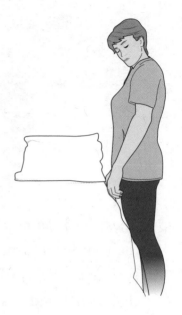

Step 5. Keeping your head turned to the side, quickly lift your head fully upright, so you are standing up with your head turned to the side (Figure 8.10). Continue to touch the chair or bed to support yourself. Another wave of dizziness might come over you. Wait until the dizziness ends before turning your head to face forward. This completes the maneuver.

After completing all the steps of the maneuver, tip your head up and down a few times. If you don't feel dizzy any longer, you may not need to do another maneuver. If you still experience a spinning sensation when you move your head, repeat the steps of the maneuver. Most people have to repeat the maneuver a few times to flush out all the particles.

Prone Half Somersault Maneuver

If you have bad back problems, and you can't tolerate bending forward to perform the seated or standing adjusted versions of the Half

Somersault maneuver just discussed, you can still do a prone version of the Half Somersault maneuver.

To perform the prone Half Somersault maneuver, complete the following steps.

Step 1. Kneel in the middle of a large bed, facing the side of the bed. Place your hands along the edge of the bed. This will help position yourself so that when you lie down on your stomach your shoulders will be at the edge of the bed. Quickly tip your head up so your eyes are looking directly at the ceiling (Figure 8.11). Look straight up, do not turn your head to either side. After doing this you might experience a few seconds of dizziness. It's OK to close your eyes but don't move or lower your head—keep it tilted up. Wait in this position for 30 seconds, or until all the spinning has stopped.

Step 2. Next, without turning your head to either side, lie down on your stomach so that your shoulders are just off the edge of the bed, but your chest is fully supported. Your head should

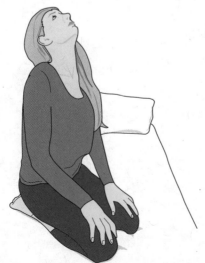

Figure 8.11   Prone Half Somersault: Step 1. Kneel on the bed with your hands along one edge. Tip your head up and back as far as possible. This may cause a brief spinning sensation.

Figure 8.12 Prone Half Somersault: Step 2. Lie down with your arms hanging down off the edge of the bed but with your chest supported on the bed. Dangle your head upside down off the side of the bed.

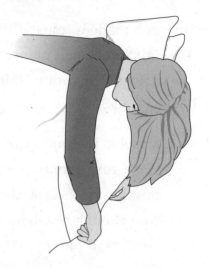

be completely off the bed. Dangle your hands down to the floor on either side of your head. Lower your head until it is hanging upside down (Figure 8.12) off the side of the bed. Once your head is upside down, you may feel spinning. Hold this position until the spinning slows or at least 30 seconds.

Step 3. Prepare to flush the particles out of the canal. To do this, turn your head so that you are looking at your elbow on the same side of your body as the problem ear (Figure 8.13). If

Figure 8.13 Prone Half Somersault: Step 3. Note that these figures illustrate treatment of the right ear. Turn your head so it is still upside down but you are looking at your right elbow.

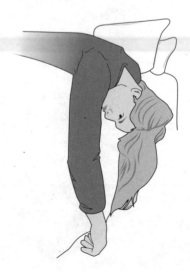

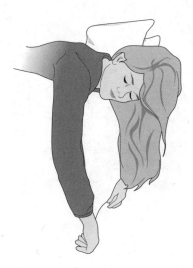

Figure 8.14   Prone Half Somersault: Step 4. Keeping your head turned to the side, quickly raise your head so it is level with your back and the bed.

the problem is with your right ear, look at your right elbow. If the problem is with your left ear, look at your left elbow. (If you are not certain, treat the right side during the first maneuver and then treat the left side with a second maneuver if you still have any symptoms.) Hold this position until all the spinning has subsided completely before moving on to the next step.

Step 4. Complete the next flushing-out step quickly. Keeping your head turned to face your elbow, quickly lift your head so it is level with your back (Figure 8.14). You might get a rush of dizziness as you do this. This is perfectly normal; just continue with the maneuver. Keep your head turned toward your elbow and level with your back and wait for the dizziness to decrease. Hold this position for about 30 seconds, until any spinning stops.

Step 5. In the final step, return to the upright position. Keeping your head turned to the side, use your legs and hands to lift your

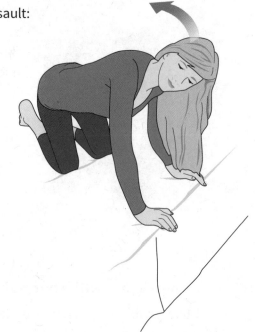

Figure 8.15 Prone Half Somersault: Step 5. Move on to your hands and knees, keeping your head level with your back, then sit back so you are kneeling with your head fully upright and turned to the side you are treating. Note that these figures illustrate treatment of the right ear.

body until you are on all fours on the bed (Figure 8.15). Once you are in this position, rock back until you are kneeling. Move your head upward, keeping it turned to the side, until it is fully upright. Another wave of dizziness might occur. Wait until all the dizziness passes before turning your head to face forward. This completes the maneuver.

After completing all the steps of the maneuver, tip your head up and down a few times. If you don't feel dizzy any longer, you may not need to do another maneuver. If you still experience a spinning sensation when you move your head, repeat the steps of the maneuver. Most people have to repeat the maneuver a few times to flush out all the particles.

Some people have more than one physical limitation, such as bad knees, a sore back, and neck stiffness. It can be difficult to move the particles by yourself if you face too many physical challenges. If this is the case, you might want to try the Semont maneuver, which is discussed in Chapter 10, "Maneuvers Performed by a Provider." Your physical therapist, primary care doctor, or ENT specialist may also be able to help with in-office maneuvers.

We've now gone over how to use the Half Somersault and its variations to resolve the most common kind of BPPV, which occurs when otoconia particles are in the posterior canal (see Chapter 3, "How Does Vertigo Happen?" if you need to review this anatomy). It is also possible to have loose particles in the other two canals, and, unfortunately, this can be a complication of doing maneuvers for posterior canal BPPV. In the next chapter, we cover treatment maneuvers to move otoconia particles that are located in the other two canals. The maneuvers covered in Chapter 9, "Unusual Forms of BPPV," are the Gufoni maneuver and the Deep Dix–Hallpike maneuver.

9

Unusual Forms of BPPV

"Anaya first noticed a little problem during her dance class. The students had all been practicing spinning in place, and she started to feel a bit tilted and wavery on her feet. The next day, while walking, she had a sudden jolt of intense spinning, but it only lasted for a couple of seconds. This happened a few more times over the course of the next few hours. That night when she rolled over in bed, she was suddenly awakened with an intense sensation of whirling. When she rolled to the opposite side, it happened again. She propped herself up on pillows and very slowly put one ear down on the pillow, and she was able to get back to sleep.

Unfortunately, on arising the next morning, Anaya staggered around her bedroom. Her head felt like it was on crooked, or as if her eyes were crossed. Any quick head movement could set off a frightful, intense spinning. Her environment spun crazily around her. She started doing a maneuver for BPPV but the dizziness was not set off by those movements. At one point, she tipped her head straight up to look at a skylight, and this set off the most violent spinning of the day, but the sensation only lasted for about 10 seconds. She called her doctor and finally

was treated for horizontal canal BPPV later that day. All the dizziness and the off-balance feeling went away and the problem
never recurred. **"**

The Half Somersault maneuver is designed to remove particles
from the posterior canal, which is the canal that is most commonly
affected by BPPV. About 90% of cases of BPPV respond to this
maneuver. Occasionally, however, crystals can migrate throughout
the labyrinth and other maneuvers are needed to resolve the resulting symptoms. The symptoms caused by these rare forms of BPPV
and the maneuvers to treat these are described in this chapter.

Any time a person has particles in a semicircular canal that move
and cause vertigo, the person can be said to have BPPV. BPPV can
affect any one (or all three) semicircular canals in either ear, and different treatments are used for each canal that is affected. Most of
the time, the particles are located in the curved arm of the posterior
semicircular canal (which is also called the inferior canal because it is
the lowest canal in the skull). The reason crystals are most often in the
posterior canal is that this canal is oriented vertically and is behind
and below the other two canals in the upright head (Figure 9.1). Since
the particles are heavy, they usually end up in the lowest part of the
ear that they can reach, which is the bottom of the posterior canal.
Once particles make it all the way down into the posterior canal, it is
quite a long way for them to travel back up in order to escape, so they
tend to build up there.

BPPV Caused by Crystals That Are Not in the Posterior Canal

In addition to the posterior canal, there are two other canals in
each ear: the horizontal canal and the anterior canal. BPPV can

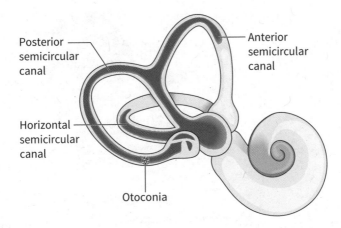

Posterior semicircular canal

Anterior semicircular canal

Horizontal semicircular canal

Otoconia

Figure 9.1 BPPV in the posterior canal. This diagram is a view of the labyrinth seen from the side. The posterior canal is furthest toward the back of the head and is the lowest canal in the ear so heavy particles tend to build up there.

occur if particles are moving in the curved part of the canal in either of these two canals (Figure 9.2 on the next page). Particles can also enter the ampulla, the enlarged bulb at one end of the canal that contains the spinning sensor, and this can affect any of the three canals. These other kinds of BPPV—where the main problem is NOT crystals moving freely in the posterior canal but crystals moving elsewhere in the ear—have different symptoms than posterior canal BPPV. Fortunately, they are rare.

How Do Crystals Get in the Other Canals?

The alternate forms of BPPV are much less common than the posterior canal form and mostly occur in people who are using maneuvers to try to treat BPPV. Everyone with BPPV has loose crystals. When doing maneuvers, the particles may fall out of the posterior canal in clumps that are perfectly sized to fit into any canal. As long you stop doing exercises as soon as the particles are all out, no problem arises.

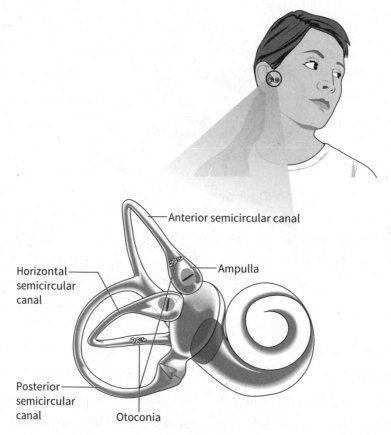

Figure 9.2   BPPV in the anterior and horizontal canals. Otoconia particles moving in these the anterior and horizontal canals can also cause vertigo attacks. If the particles enter the ampulla, the symptoms change and the treatment is more difficult.

However, what if you're not sure they are all out? What if you do one more exercise just to be sure?

Putting your head back and upside down for one more of these maneuvers means that any particles that have been successfully moved back where they belong are now right above the openings that lead back into the canals. If a perfectly canal-sized chunk of particles is right beside that opening, it is perfectly positioned to fall back into any of the canals.

The Half Somersault maneuver is designed to prevent this complication by having you bend forward instead of lying back. Unfortunately, most other maneuvers require you to tilt your head backward and dangle it and that makes it more likely that the particles will fall into another canal. This happens most often when the head is tipped far back during the Dix–Hallpike maneuver (see Chapter 2, "The History of BPPV," p. 20). The Dix–Hallpike is the start of many maneuvers, such as the Epley and Semont maneuvers. If you have just completed a previous maneuver, and then decide to try one more time, particles are especially likely to switch canals.[1] The indication that a just-removed particle is falling back into a canal is a sudden change in the dizziness. Your head may feel like it's spinning in a different (opposite or reversed) direction, and the dizziness tends to be much more severe. If this happens to you, one of the easiest and most effective things to do is to sit back up and wait for at least half an hour before attempting any more maneuvers. This may stop the problem because the particles fall right back out when you sit up. However, it can be difficult to remember to do this when you are very dizzy. If you don't immediately sit up, or if you sit up too slowly, the particles may remain in the anterior or horizontal canals. In that case, it may be necessary to do the other maneuvers described in this chapter to clear out particles that have entered these other canals too deeply.

The Horizontal Canal and H-BPPV

The horizontal canal is along the horizontal plane in the head, tilted slightly upward at the front (Figure 9.3 on the next page). Particles can travel into this canal when doing the Dix–Hallpike maneuver, when you make very quick head turns when upright (as Anaya

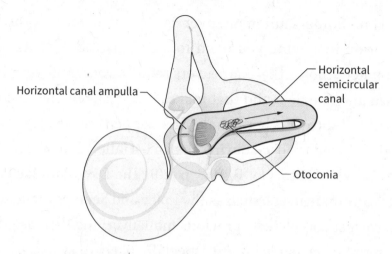

Horizontal canal ampulla

Horizontal semicircular canal

Otoconia

Figure 9.3   BPPV of the horizontal canal. In the example illustrated here, the otoconia particles have rolled to the end of the canal that is blocked by the ampulla. They cannot roll out on their own because the canal has an upward tilt and to roll out, the otoconia would have to roll uphill.

noticed in the chapter-opening story), or when you are lying on one side. Turning the head from side to side when you are upright moves the fluid in the horizontal canal. This allows any misplaced particles that are inside this canal to roll out on their own in most cases. However, if there are a large number of particles in the horizontal canal, and if they move all the way around the canal to the end that is blocked by the sensor, the movement can cause dizziness so severe that the afflicted person will go to any length to avoid movement of the head.[2] If the head isn't moved enough, the particles don't roll out of the horizontal canal and they can keep causing severe dizziness.

BPPV in the horizontal canal (*H-BPPV*) affects people very differently from the usual posterior canal variety. It is much, much more violent and nauseating. As noted previously, H-BPPV can begin while doing maneuvers to dislodge crystals from the posterior canal, but it also can occasionally begin when a person is simply rolling over in bed. Most of the time, however, it is triggered by the movements of the Dix–Hallpike maneuver.[3]

We use the horizontal canal constantly as we move around because we turn our head frequently from side to side. The head movements we make in the horizontal plane last longer than those we make vertically. For example, when you look up at a cloud, you tip your head less than 90 degrees and the movement takes only a second. In contrast, when turning about-face, you move 180 degrees horizontally and this takes correspondingly longer. Our brains accordingly pay more attention to the sensation of movement coming from the horizontal canal and the feeling of movement tends to last longer from this canal than from the other two canals. If particles happen to enter this more-sensitive canal, the dizziness is intense. This is the type of BPPV that affected Anaya in the chapter-opening story.

The horizontal canal is responsible for making eye movements from side to side. Look at yourself in a mirror, and then turn your head slowly to the right and left while looking at your pupils. You will see them move from the corner of the eye to the opposite corner as you move back and forth. This movement is being generated by your horizontal canals. If you suffer from BPPV in the horizontal canal, this same horizontal eye movement happens, but it is much faster. The eyes scan across horizontally, and then jerk back, scan and jerk back. You will see the room spin horizontally in a blur. To see what horizontal nystagmus looks like, close your eyes and spin in place. After a minute or two of spinning, open your eyes. You will have a horizontal nystagmus. If you try to focus on a light, you will see it repeatedly pass by in a horizontal streak.

If you have H-BPPV and hold perfectly still with your head upright, it will gradually die down, but it might take a couple of minutes for the vertigo to go away completely. Once the vertigo has died down, turning your head from side to side, especially while you are lying down, can set it off again. The most unpleasant part is that this kind of vertigo and horizontal nystagmus is exceptionally nauseating. It's normal to begin vomiting within 30 to 60 seconds after it starts.

Another characteristic of H-BPPV is that the direction of spinning can reverse. If you notice the world spinning to the right when lying on your right side, but it spins to the left when you lie on your left side, it is a good indicator that you have H-BPPV. However, this reversal can also happen to patients in a few unrelated vertigo disorders and so is not absolutely diagnostic.

If you have just completed a Dix–Hallpike maneuver when you start to feel the symptoms of H-BPPV, the best thing to do is to immediately sit up. Often the particles will fall right back out and the H-BPPV spell will stop. If the dizziness does not go away, there are special maneuvers designed to remove the crystals from the horizontal canal. Often it is necessary to visit a trained therapist—either a physical therapist, an audiologist, or an ENT doctor who is familiar with maneuvers. However, we also discuss how to do these maneuvers yourself later in this chapter.

Many inner ear diseases besides BPPV result in horizontal nystagmus, but the vertigo and nystagmus they cause is usually different than the kind caused by H-BPPV. In those non-BPPV diseases, the horizontal nystagmus doesn't die away completely when the head is held perfectly still and upright. In these other disorders, even if the dizziness subsides when sitting, it can often be reignited by just turning the eyes to one side or the other when the head is perfectly still. If you experience this, these are signs you do not have H-BPPV. See Chapter 4, "Non-BPPV Causes of Vertigo," and Chapter 5, "Central

Vertigo: Non-BPPV Positional Vertigo and Nystagmus" for other causes of vertigo that are not BPPV.

The Anterior Canal and A-BPPV

The third canal is the anterior canal. It is also called the superior canal because it is the highest canal in the ear. The arch of the anterior canal is located in front of and above the openings to all of the canals in the inner ear (Figure 9.4). Because the entire anterior canal is above the opening, when the head is upright, otoconia particles cannot move into it by gravity. Particles enter the anterior canal when the head is upside down, but when the head is moved upright again, they usually fall right back out. The only time the source of BPPV is in this canal and people experience *A-BPPV* is if particles fall in when the head is upside down and the head is subsequently

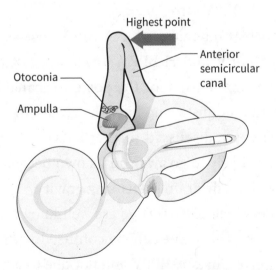

Highest point

Anterior semicircular canal

Otoconia

Ampulla

Figure 9.4 BPPV of the anterior canal. Particles that enter the anterior canal will fall back out when the head is upright unless they have gone past the point marked by the arrow. Any particles that move past that point fall down and become lodged in or near the ampulla.

rotated even further vertically so that the particles move beyond the halfway point of the canal's curve. After this series of events has happened, when the head is raised, the crystals can fall down towards the sensor and pile up there. Crystals in the anterior canal are found in only about two of a hundred patients with BPPV.[4] In short, it's fairly difficult to get particles deep enough into the anterior canal to cause ongoing symptoms.

The primary symptom of A-BPPV is vertical nystagmus.[5] When you experience vertical nystagmus, the world looks like it is rolling downward not unlike what you may see if you scroll too fast down on a computer screen. A-BPPV can happen when lying down with the head turned, but even lying down face down without turning the head can set off A-BPPV. It tends to come on suddenly just like posterior canal BPPV. And also like posterior canal BPPV, A-BPPV goes away if the head is held upright and not moving. Tilting the head up or down can set A-BPPV off again.

There are special maneuvers for A-BPPV just as there are for posterior canal BPPV and H-BPPV. These are not as commonly performed as the maneuvers for the posterior canal and so it can be hard to locate therapists who have the ability to perform these. A-BPPV exercises are discussed further later this chapter. Fortunately, A-BPPV is likely to go away on its own because much of the anterior canal can easily drain itself using gravity.

Brain disorders that cause vertigo are well-known to cause vertical nystagmus, and this can easily be confused with A-BPPV. The signs that your problem is A-BPPV and not due to a problem in the brain is that A-BPPV usually begins after an attack of posterior canal BPPV, especially if you have been doing maneuvers. If you have A-BPPV, the illusion of vertical scrolling lasts for less than a minute before stopping. In contrast, vertical nystagmus that stems from brain problems can last as long as the position that triggers the nystagmus is held.

Ampullary BPPV: Crystals in or near the Ampulla

Each semicircular canal is about three-quarters of a circle, with an opening to the inner ear near the gravity sensor at one end and a closed spinning sensor at the other end. Particles can move all the way around the curve until they reach the spinning sensor, which is contained in the ampulla, an enlarged bulb at one end of the canal. The junction between the large ampulla and the narrow canal is shaped like a funnel (Figure 9.5 on the next page).

If particles accumulate in the ampulla and then stick together, they can form a ball of particles that is larger than the canal and cause *ampullary BPPV.* Try to pour sugar quickly through a funnel. You will notice that it tends to get blocked; eventually you have to tap it to get the sugar running again. The same thing can happen with otoconia in people with *ampullary BPPV.* A ball of otoconia can become trapped within the ampulla because it is too large to exit back to the canal. The ball of particles acts like a tiny ball-valve in the opening from the ampulla to the canal. Normally fluid moves through the opening whenever the head is turned, allowing the sensor to move. However, if there is a ball-valve of particles in the opening, movement of fluid pushes the ball into the opening and shuts off the flow of fluid, disabling the canal's sensor (Figure 9.6 on p. 139).[6]

It is also believed that there may be narrow parts of the canal near the ampulla that can be the site of traffic jams of crystals. When these traffic jams occur, the symptoms are the same as having particles trapped in the ampulla. This complication, called canalith jam,

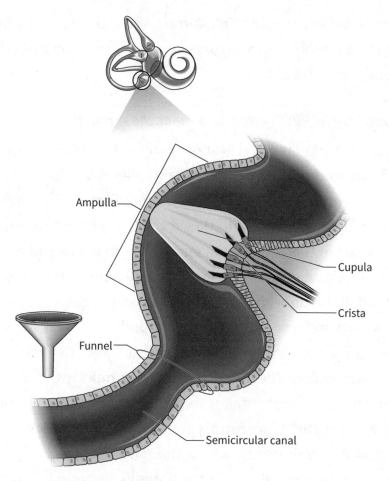

Ampulla

Cupula

Crista

Funnel

Semicircular canal

Figure 9.5   The spinning sensor of the inner ear. The crista is a ridge with the cupula on the top. The cupula completely seals off the ampulla so particles cannot exit past it. The only way otoconia crystals can exit the ampulla is by going back out the way they came in, back into the canal, but this exit is funnel-shaped. If a cluster of otoconia forms in the ampulla that is larger than the canal, the particles will not be able to exit.

is treated the same as ampullary BPPV. Crystals are also believed to occasionally adhere to the cupula in the ampulla, so that the cupula is turned into a gravity sensor. This is called cupulolithiasis and is another form of ampullary BPPV.

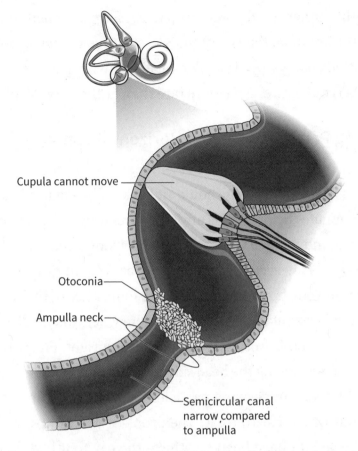

Cupula cannot move

Otoconia

Ampulla neck

Semicircular canal
narrow compared
to ampulla

Figure 9.6   Otoconia jammed in the canal. A large ball of otoconia crystals can lodge in the funnel where the ampulla joins the canal or in a narrow segment of the canal. This prevents fluid movement and shuts off the canal sensor causing ampullary BPPV.

In ampullary BPPV caused by ball-valving particles, the canal acts like it has been shut off. The key symptom is persistent nystagmus. Nystagmus is horizontal if the problem is in the horizontal canal; down-beating if the problem is in the posterior canal; and upbeating if it is in the anterior canal. Nystagmus is triggered by head movement, but it lasts much longer than nystagmus in regular BPPV and is easily mistaken for nystagmus from a brain disease such as a tumor or stroke, or another inner ear disorder. If particles are attached to the sensor inside the ampulla, the symptom is nystagmus that changes direction as the head changes position. Fortunately, having particles stuck in the ampulla is quite rare, even more rare than H-BPPV or A-BPPV.

Clearing Particles from the Horizontal Canal

If you perform a Dix–Hallpike maneuver and you suddenly see the room spinning horizontally, you should sit back up immediately and wait at least 15 minutes before trying any maneuver movement again to reduce the risk of moving particles into the horizontal semicircular canal a second time. However, if you do not get back up in time, particles may fall deep in your horizontal canal. The indication of this is seeing the room spin horizontally for up to a minute when you lie down or when you turn your head from side to side when upright. Frequent vomiting brought on by moving the head side to side is also an indication.

The first step in clearing particles from the horizontal canal is to figure out which ear to treat. The problem will almost always be in the ear that you have been treating—the ear that had the posterior canal BPPV. If you were working on your right ear when the new problem arose, you should do maneuvers for BPPV caused by crystals in the horizontal canal (H-BPPV) of the right ear. If you were not certain which ear had the problem, do one maneuver for each ear. Several different maneuvers have been created for BPPV caused by crystals in the horizontal canal (H-BPPV), but the most effective one is the *Gufoni maneuver* named after its creator Dr. Mauro Gufoni of Livorno, Italy, who devised it in 1998.[7] The version we present here has been slightly modified to more effectively help move particles out of the horizontal canal.

To perform the Gufoni maneuver follow these steps:

Step 1. Sit facing outward on the edge of the bed (Figure 9.7 on the next page).

Step 2. To treat the right ear, turn your head about halfway to your shoulder to the right

Step 3. Tip over onto your left side, so you end up on your side with your left shoulder down and your head looking up at the ceiling (Figure 9.8 on the next page). You may experience a strong spinning sensation while in this position. Don't move; just allow the spinning to take place. It will die down after several seconds or a minute. Wait at least 30 seconds in this position, or until the severe spinning comes to a stop.

Step 4. Staying on your left side, slowly turn your head toward the left shoulder until you are facing the bed. Your head will be turned completely toward your left shoulder at this point (Figure 9.9 on the next page). Hold this position until all spinning stops or for a full minute.

Step 5. The final step is to sit back up (Figure 9.10 on page 143). Keeping your head turned fully to the left shoulder, push yourself upright by swinging your shoulders in an arc to the right. Once you are fully upright, try moving your head from side to side. If no vertigo occurs, you can stop doing maneuvers.

Figure 9.7   Gufoni maneuver, treatment of the right ear: Steps 1 and 2. Sit on the edge of the bed. Turn your head to the right about halfway to the shoulder.

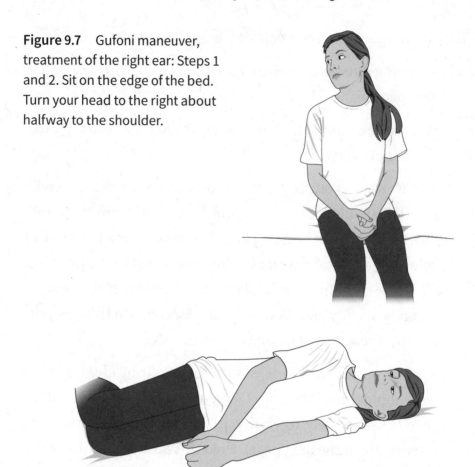

Figure 9.8   Gufoni maneuver, treatment of the right ear: Step 3. Keeping your head turned to the right, fall straight over onto your side with your left shoulder down. You will end up facing the ceiling.

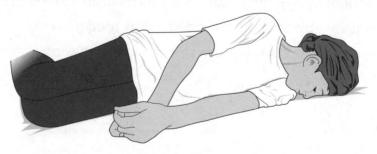

Figure 9.9   Gufoni maneuver, treatment of the right ear: Step 4. Turn your head to the left slowly, until you are first facing straight ahead and then facing the bed.

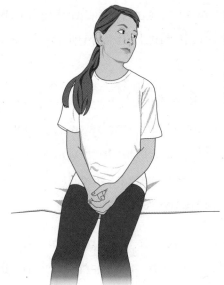

Figure 9.10   Gufoni maneuver, treatment of the right ear: Step 5. Sit up while keeping your head turned to the left. Once you are upright, turn your head back to the center.

If your problem is in the left ear, or if you continue to have symptoms after a couple of right-sided Gufoni maneuvers, treat the left ear. To do so, follow these steps (Figure 9.11 on the next page):

Step 1. Sit facing outward on the edge of the bed for this maneuver.

Step 2. To treat the left ear, turn your head about halfway to your shoulder to the left.

Step 3. Then tip over on your right side, so you end up on your side with your right shoulder down and your head looking up at the ceiling. You may experience a strong spinning sensation while in this position. (Figure 9.12 page 145). Don't move; just allow the spinning to take place. It will die down after several seconds or a minute. Wait at least 30 seconds in this position, or until the severe spinning comes to a stop.

Step 4. Staying on your right side, slowly turn your head toward the right shoulder until you are facing the bed. Your head will be turned completely toward your right shoulder at this point (Figure 9.13). Again, wait until all spinning stops or for a full minute.

Step 5. The final step is to sit back up. Keeping your head turned fully to the right shoulder, push yourself upright by swinging your torso in an arc to the left (Figure 9.14). Once you are fully upright, try moving your head from side to side. If no vertigo occurs, you can stop doing maneuvers.

You may need to repeat the maneuver. If the problem did not resolve the first time, make an extra effort to hold each position for a full minute.

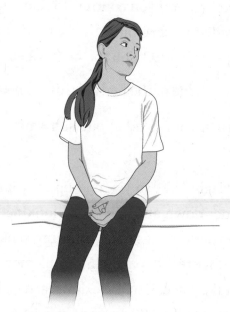

Figure 9.11   Gufoni maneuver, treatment of the left ear: Steps 1 and 2. Sit on the edge of the bed. Turn your head to the left about halfway to the shoulder.

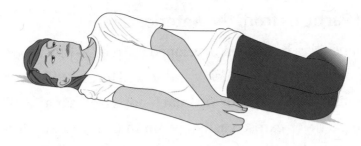

Figure 9.12   Gufoni maneuver, treatment of the left ear: Step 3. Keeping your head turned to the right, fall straight over onto your side with your right shoulder down. You will end up facing the ceiling.

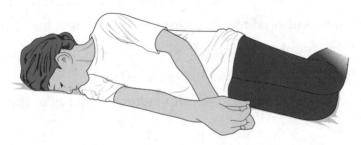

Figure 9.13   Gufoni maneuver, treatment of the left ear: Step 4. Turn your head to the right slowly, until you are first facing straight ahead and then facing the bed.

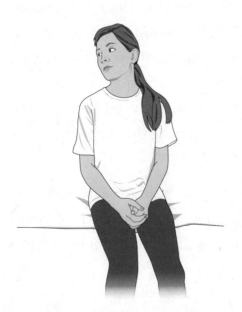

Figure 9.14   Gufoni maneuver, treatment of the left ear: Step 5. Sit up while keeping your head turned to the right. Once you are upright, turn your head back to the center.

Clearing Particles from the Anterior Canal

Several maneuvers have been developed to treat A-BPPV, but in general, none of these work as quickly and as well for A-BPPV as the Epley or Half Somersault work for ordinary posterior canal BPPV. This is because particles can so easily end up in the ampulla in A-BPPV, where they tend to become trapped. The *"Deep" Dix–Hallpike maneuver* is the simplest maneuver to use at home to treat A-BPPV. This modification of the Dix–Hallpike maneuver was devised by Drs. Dario Yacovino, Timothy Hain, and Francisco Gualtieri in 2009,[8] but we have made additional modifications in this book. One of the nice features of this maneuver is that it works for both anterior canals, so you don't have to worry about which side to treat.

To perform the "Deep" Dix–Hallpike maneuver, take the following steps:

Step 1. Lie down on your back on a bed so that your head dangles off the edge backward. Try to place yourself so that your head is nearly upside down (Figure 9.15). Hold this position for about a minute or until all the spinning stops. You can help mobilize the particles by tapping with your fingertip on the bone behind your ear or putting something that vibrates against that area. Even a vibrating electric toothbrush handle pressed behind the ear can help during this step if particles are trapped in the ampulla.

Step 2. Next, tip your chin down and your head forward and prop yourself up on your elbows so that you are facing upward and forward (Figure 9.16). We call this the Beach Position. Stay in this position for a minute.

Step 3. Next sit up all the way, facing straight forward. Then continue moving in a forward arc until your face almost touches your knee (Figure 9.17 on the next page). Wait for a minute, and then sit upright.

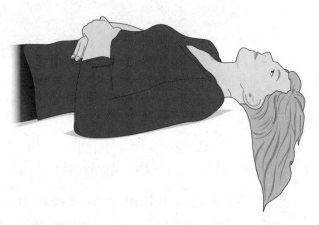

Figure 9.15   Deep Dix–Hallpike: Step 1. This exercise treats the anterior canal of both ears. Hang your head off the side edge of the bed.

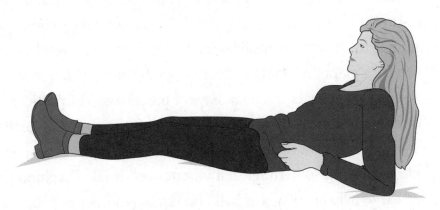

Figure 9.16   Deep Dix–Hallpike: Step 2 ("Beach Position"). Sit partway up and lean back on your elbows as you would if you were lying on a beach looking at the ocean. Then tip your head back slightly so you are looking toward the intersection of a wall and the ceiling.

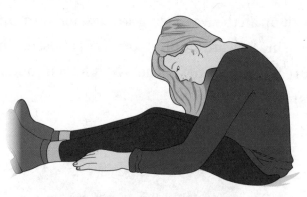

Figure 9.17 Deep Dix–Hallpike: Step 3. Sit up and continue moving forward until your nose touches your knee or your face is completely horizontal and facing downward.

Clearing Particles from the Ampulla

Vibration and tapping can help particles exit the ampulla, but it can take a great deal of work to break up a large ball-valve obstruction or to remove particles from the cupula. Once particles are stuck in an ampulla, the usual maneuvers do not work because the particles are no longer in the canal. It is necessary to break up the clump first, and then to perform the maneuvers for that canal. The easiest way to break up the clump is to shake your head back and forth briskly several times, and then try a maneuver for the affected canal. You will likely need to do this several times a day for a few days or more to get the particles to exit the ampulla. Once all the particles have left the ampulla, further maneuvers can remove them from the canal. A therapist or assistant can help by placing something that vibrates on the skull behind the affected ear to help break up the ball of crystals. Another way to break up the particles is to use a variation of the *Semont maneuver*, which is outlined step-by-step in Chapter 10, "Maneuvers Performed by a Provider." Start seated on the side of a bed, then tip over onto one shoulder rather roughly. Keep facing straight forward; do not turn the head as is done during the Semont maneuver. As quickly as possible, sit back up and swing over until you are lying on the other shoulder. By moving back and forth briskly, you can sometimes shake the particles loose into the canal; this is heralded by a sudden wave of spinning. Then do the Half Somersault, the Deep Dix–Hallpike, or if the spinning is horizontal, use the Gufoni maneuver to remove the dislodged particles from the canal.

As you have learned, there are many maneuvers for BPPV. We've covered the most effective maneuvers for the horizontal and anterior canals in this chapter. You may have had other maneuvers done by a therapist or have been given different exercises to do at home. The next chapter discusses the most common alternate exercises and complications to avoid.

10

Maneuvers Performed by a Provider

"Anton, a retiree and avid golfer, awakened one morning to find his bedroom spinning. The vertigo struck when he rolled over in bed, so in an effort to make it stop, he rolled immediately in the other direction. The spinning stopped after a few seconds. He felt better sitting in a recliner instead of lying down, so he stayed there until his head felt more settled. He felt much better once he was up and around, but when he tried golfing, the symptoms flared up again. When he leaned over to put in a tee, he could feel a little spin that worsened when he stood back up. After weeks of this, Anton became very discouraged and considered giving up golfing. His primary care doctor was not certain what was causing the problem and had him see a cardiologist, but all the tests they gave him came out fine. He was eventually seen by a vertigo specialist and was found to have BPPV. Three Epley maneuvers were done in one sitting, and his dizziness completely disappeared. He was able to resume golfing without any symptoms."

We've introduced you to the simplest and most effective home exercises for BPPV in all three canals in the preceding chapters. If you have had BPPV in the past, you may have already been seen by a physician, physical therapist, or audiologist to have maneuvers performed by them. Sometimes these maneuvers are given out as home exercises, but for most people, the maneuvers we cover in this chapter have limitations as home exercises. Some providers also still use maneuvers that are obsolete or not highly effective and are simply not helpful for home use. In this chapter, we summarize maneuvers that we have not covered elsewhere in the book that are often used by providers and discuss complications to watch for if you try these at home.

The Dix–Hallpike Maneuver

The first step in treating BPPV is to diagnose it, and the Dix–Hallpike maneuver is the standard method to do this (see Chapter 2, "The History of BPPV," p. 20). With the exception of the Half Somersault, almost all maneuvers begin with a version of the Dix–Hallpike maneuver. The Dix–Hallpike maneuver maximizes nystagmus and makes it easy for the provider, who has a full view of the patient's face during the maneuver, to identify which ear has the problem. Once the Dix–Hallpike maneuver is performed, the particles in the posterior semicircular canal of the ear will have rotated nearly halfway around the canal, so only a little more needs to be done to complete the removal of particles. For these reasons, starting treatment with the Dix–Hallpike maneuver is very efficient for clinicians.

However, the Dix–Hallpike is *not* the best way to begin if you are trying to perform any maneuver by yourself at home. The Dix–Hallpike maneuver actually makes your dizziness as intense as possible. The head movement moves the crystals toward the exit of the canal at the same time that the fluid in the canal is moving violently in the same direction. This maximizes the speed of particle movement, so the nystagmus is made more dramatic. That's good if an observer, like a doctor, is trying to see nystagmus, but it is not so good for the sufferer, who can be so frightened or sickened that they can't continue to execute the maneuver.

All maneuvers that begin with the Dix–Hallpike maneuver have another risk: Particles that have been removed can fall back in when the next Dix–Hallpike maneuver is done.[1] This is referred to as *reflux* of otoconia. At the conclusion of any successful Dix–Hallpike maneuver, there are particles that have been molded into a mass that fits perfectly in the canals that are now lying just outside the entrances to the canals. If you do another Dix–Hallpike, your head will be put in a position that places this heavy mass of particles right above the entrances to the canals. As you lie down, any particles near those openings can move toward the openings and get pushed right into the canals because the fluid movement forces them in exactly that direction (Figure 10.1 on the next page). The two canals most likely to be affected by this reflux of crystals are the posterior and horizontal canals, and both are affected about equally. You learn more about BPPV in these canals in Chapter 9, "Unusual Forms of BPPV."

The safest way to avoid this complication is to wait at least 15 minutes between maneuvers so that the particles have time to drift farther away from the opening before the next Dix–Hallpike maneuver is done. Waiting also allows you to see if you feel better after the first maneuver. If your vertigo is gone, there is no need to do another.

If you do encounter this problem, you may notice that the spinning after the Dix–Hallpike seems to be more severe or your head seems to be spinning in a new direction. If this occurs, the treatment is very simple: You must sit back up to stop the maneuver as soon as the problem occurs. This allows any particles that are entering the canals to exit before they move too far into the canal and get stuck there. However, this only works if you recognize what is happening. Without someone

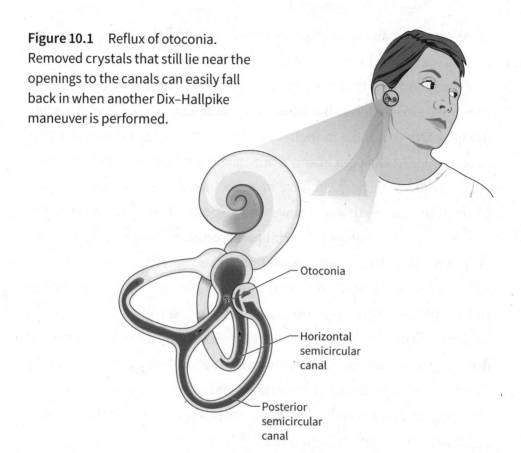

Figure 10.1   Reflux of otoconia. Removed crystals that still lie near the openings to the canals can easily fall back in when another Dix–Hallpike maneuver is performed.

Otoconia

Horizontal semicircular canal

Posterior semicircular canal

to watch their eye movements and to help them decide if there is a problem, people tend to wait too long and lose the few seconds of opportunity to fix the problem. It is difficult even for a "spotter" to notice this quickly enough, especially if you close your eyes because the dizziness is so severe. For these reasons, the exercises that include the Dix–Hallpike are best used with a trained provider to assist you.

The Epley Maneuver

The Epley maneuver is the maneuver that is most commonly used by clinicians and therapists to treat BPPV.[2] A few minor variations of this maneuver have been made, but the basic movements are similar for most versions. The Epley maneuver makes nystagmus easy for the observer to see, so the location of the displaced particles can be identified, and it rotates the particles smoothly around the posterior canal toward the exit without sloshing them back and forth. It is ideal for use in the clinic because it begins with the Dix–Hallpike, allowing the diagnosis to be made and the treatment to be applied in one maneuver. Also, the provider has a clear view of the nystagmus during the Dix–Hallpike because the patient is facing up.

The Epley maneuver is usually performed on a reclining chair or narrow table. One or two people are needed to view the nystagmus, help the patient move properly, and prevent the patient from falling off the table or bed. It is safest to use two people, one on each side of a narrow table, so that they can prevent any falls during the procedure.

In the Epley maneuver, the patient sits lengthwise on the exam table, facing the end of the table (Figure 10.2). The patient should be seated close enough to the head of the table so that, when the patient lies down, the shoulders are on the table but the head extends beyond it. The clinician begins on the same side of the bed as the problem

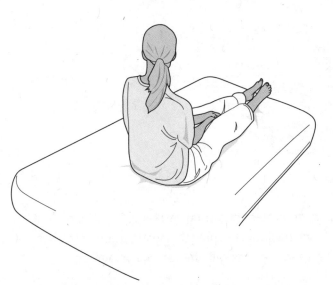

Figure 10.2 Epley maneuver, treatment of the left ear: Beginning position. The patient is seated with the head turned about 45 degrees toward the left shoulder.

ear. If the patient reports dizziness when rolling over to the right, for example, then the clinician will stand on the patient's right side.

The clinician grasps the sides of the patient's head with two hands and turns the head until the patient is facing the clinician with their head turned at about a 45-degree angle from the centerline of the bed. The clinician should hold the head firmly so that the neck will not be torqued or twisted during the maneuver. I ask the patient to grasp my elbow that is closest to the table with one or both hands to add stability and allow the patient to feel more secure during the procedure. It is optimal if patients keep their eyes open even when dizziness occurs, so that the nystagmus can be seen clearly. The patient is made to lie back very quickly, keeping the head turned to the side at 45 degrees, until flat on the back with the head supported by the clinician's hands just off the end of the table (Figure 10.3). The clinician then allows the patient's head to tip back further with the chin upward so that the top of the head is below the surface of the

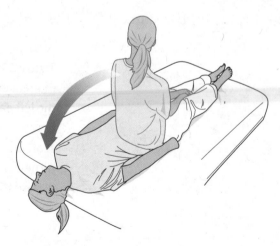

Figure 10.3   Epley maneuver, treatment of the left ear: Lying flat. The patient is quickly moved to the reclining position, keeping the head turned to the left. This triggers a burst of vertigo and the eyes will often show nystagmus.

table. Usually within a few seconds the dizziness and corresponding nystagmus begin. Patients often report a strong sensation of falling from the table and need to hold on to the clinician's elbow tightly until the wave of vertigo passes. The affected ear is down and the normal ear is up in this position.

Once the spinning feeling and nystagmus has completely passed, the clinician will help the patient rotate on the table. The rotation is always away from the bad ear (Figure 10.4). For example, if the bad ear is the left ear, patients will lie down with the head turned to their left side, so the left ear is downward when they are reclining, and the next move is to help the patient roll to the right. In this case, the clinician instructs the patient to turn their head toward their right shoulder while the clinician guides the head to face about a 45-degree angle to the right. The clinician pauses here for at least 30

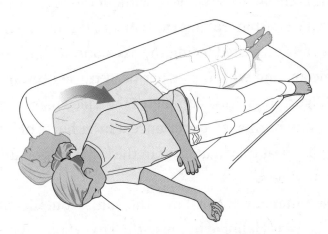

Figure 10.4 Epley maneuver, treatment of the left ear: Head turned. The patient's head is turned 90 degrees to the right and movement is paused for 30 seconds. The head is then moved another 90 degrees while the patient is helped to roll up on their right shoulder so that the patient ends up on their right side, facing downward towards the floor at a 45-degree angle.

second to allow any dizziness to pass. Then, keeping the head stable on the neck and shoulders, the clinician has an assistant on the other side of the table grasp the patient's left hand and pull them up onto their right side. Since the head started at a 45-degree angle toward the right shoulder at the beginning of this step, this means the person is now facing the floor on the right side of the table at a 45-degree angle. The clinician can again pause here to wait for the particles to settle. When the vertigo and nystagmus cease, it is an indication that the particles have settled.

At this point the patient is lying on their right side facing the assistant. The clinician is on the opposite side of the table, behind the patient's back. The clinician is holding the patient's head from the back, one hand on each side over the ears. The clinician asks the patient to move his or her legs off the table as if he or she were about to sit up facing the assistant. The patient is then instructed to sit up quickly. The clinician lifts the head without moving the head on the neck, while the assistant rotates the patient's legs off the table so that the patient ends up seated facing the assistant, with his or her back to the clinician, and with his or her head turned toward the right shoulder. (Figure 10.5) This completes the Epley maneuver. At each movement, it is normal to experience a brief burst of vertigo. The clinician will repeat this maneuver in the same session until there is no further dizziness.

The Epley maneuver can have the same complications listed above for the Dix–Hallpike because the Dix–Hallpike maneuver is the first step in the Epley maneuver. Another complication of the Epley maneuver is a tendency for the particles to roll back to the bottom of the canal when the patient is moved to the final, sitting-up position, rather than moving forward and exiting. Sometimes the

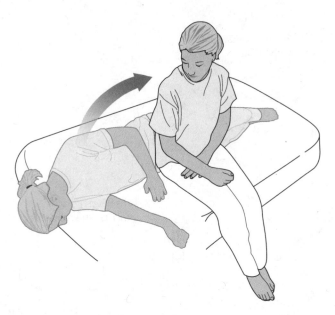

Figure 10.5   Epley maneuver, treatment of the left ear: Sitting up. While the patient's head is kept turned to the right shoulder, the patient is assisted to a seated position on the side of the table or bed.

crystals don't make it all the way to the exit during the maneuver, and if they start to fall back down into the canal instead of coming out, it makes the dizziness suddenly return with a vengeance.

When I perform this maneuver on my patients, I change the ending of this maneuver to make this complication less likely. I have patients tuck their chin down to look at the floor when moving to the sitting position in the final step of the Epley maneuver. This adjustment makes particles that are near the exit less likely to accidentally roll back down into the canal (Figure 10.6(1) on the next page). Then I turn the head 45 degrees toward the affected side and quickly move the head upright (Figures 10.6(2) and 10.6(3)). This helps flush out any particles that are teetering on the edge and at risk of falling back into the canal.

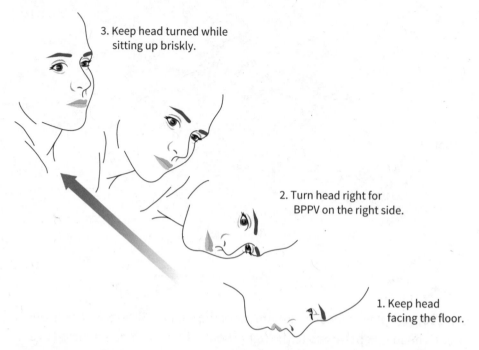

3. Keep head turned while sitting up briskly.

2. Turn head right for BPPV on the right side.

1. Keep head facing the floor.

Figure 10.6   Foster modifications of Epley maneuver. (1) When lifting the patient back to upright (see Figure 10.5), keep the patient's head down so they are leaning forward facing the floor. (2) Rotate the head 45 degrees to the right if treating the right ear (pictured) or to the left if treating the left ear. (3) Then the provider should quickly pull the patient's head and shoulders back until the head is upright. Note that the head does not snap back; instead the entire body is moved back while the head and neck are kept stable and turned throughout toward the affected side.

The Epley maneuver is difficult to do without assistance because the traditional Dix–Hallpike involves dangling your head off the end of the bed, and you have to flip yourself backward to do this. It's not a good idea to snap your neck back without support. During the Epley maneuver in a clinic, a provider stabilizes your head and neck and supports your head when it is off the bed. This is not possible when attempting to do this maneuver alone. It is safer to have someone who can help you by supporting your head as you lie back. The Half Somersault maneuver is a safer alternative for home treatment. For step-by-step instructions on how to perform the Half Somersault maneuver, review Chapter 7, "The Half Somersault Maneuver."

The Semont Maneuver

Like the Epley maneuver, the Semont maneuver is also effective when performed in a clinical setting. However, the Semont is not as effective as the Epley maneuver because the movements of the Semont maneuver do not rotate the particles continuously around the canal toward the exit; instead, when the Semont maneuver is performed the crystals are sloshed back and forth a bit. This means it is possible for some crystals to travel deeper into the canal instead of exiting.

However, if performed until all the dizziness stops, the Semont maneuver still has a very high success rate at clearing particles. The Semont maneuver also has an advantage over the Epley maneuver: It is performed with the patient sitting on the side of an exam table facing the clinician, so it can be done by a single provider without an assistant and does not require a narrow table. A bed, couch, or exam table of any width can be used.

Like the Epley maneuver, the Semont maneuver begins with a version of the Dix–Hallpike maneuver. The Dix–Hallpike portion of the Semont maneuver ends with the patient's affected ear down at a 45-degree angle to the affected side, just as in the Epley maneuver. However, the body is moved in a different way during the Semont maneuver than it is in the ordinary Dix–Hallpike maneuver. In the Semont maneuver, the patient sits on the edge of the bed facing the clinician, and the clinician holds the patient's head with both hands. The head is rotated 45 degrees *away* from the bad ear. In this example we will use the right ear as the problematic one. The head is rotated halfway toward the left shoulder. The patient is then tipped over onto the right shoulder (the shoulder on the same side as the bad ear). Note that this places the patient on his or her side, but the head is in the same position as it is during the regular Dix–Hallpike maneuver: tipped back with the right ear down (Figure 10.7). Because the head is cushioned by the bed, however, the head does not dangle as far upside down as it does during a regular Dix–Hallpike maneuver and so the particles do not make it quite as far around the canal as they do in the Epley maneuver. The nystagmus and dizziness the patient

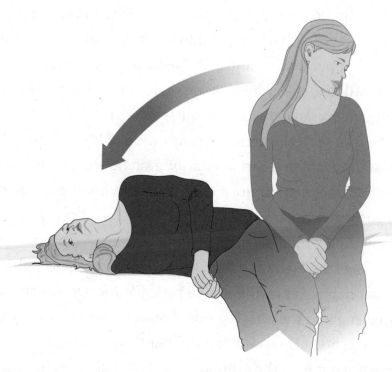

Figure 10.7 Semont maneuver, treatment of the right ear. The patient is seated on the edge of a bed. The head is turned halfway to the left shoulder. The patient is tipped over onto the right shoulder so they end up lying on their right side. The head is turned to face upward.

experiences are similar to what they feel during the Dix–Hallpike and Epley maneuvers. The Semont maneuver is paused at this point while the patient and clinician wait for the particles to settle.

Once all nystagmus has passed, keeping the head turned toward the left shoulder (the opposite shoulder from the bad ear), the patient is swung to the upright seated position and then rolled smoothly down onto his or her other side, so that the left shoulder is now on the bed and the head is facing 45 degrees downward toward the floor (Figure 10.8). At the start of this movement, fluid in the canal sloshes back in the opposite direction, which can move the particles back inward instead of out, but by the time the patient is on the other shoulder, any

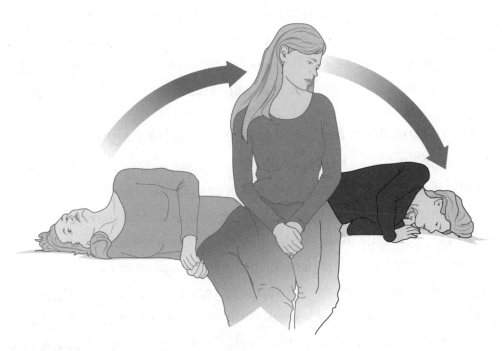

Figure 10.8   Semont maneuver, treatment of the right ear. Keeping the head turned to the left, the patient is raised to upright and then smoothly moved to a position with the left shoulder down. The head will be facing the bed. After at least 30 seconds, the patient is raised to the upright seated position.

particles that are more than halfway around the ring of the canal are in a perfect position to fall out. The patient is held in this position for 30 seconds or until the dizziness has entirely subsided and then is raised upright, which serves to push any teetering particles out and clear of the canal. Like the Epley maneuver, the Semont maneuver is repeated until all particles have exited and no further dizziness occurs.

Like all maneuvers that include the Dix–Hallpike, there is a risk of severe dizziness, and reentry of the particles into a canal when maneuvers are repeated can still occur. The Semont maneuver's version of the Dix–Hallpike doesn't allow the head to dangle like the Epley maneuver so it is safer to do by yourself, but the particles also don't go quite as far around the canal during the first step because of that, and so it may take more tries to remove all of the offending particles. As mentioned in Chapter 8, "Variations of the Half Somersault Maneuver," the Semont maneuver can be a good alternative for people with bad knees and backs, since it doesn't require kneeling or flexing the back.

Other Maneuvers for BPPV in the Posterior Canal

In Chapter 2, "The History of BPPV," we discussed older maneuvers that are still shared with patients occasionally. The Cawthorne–Cooksey exercises, for example, have been used for 80 years, but they are not specifically designed for BPPV. The Cawthorne exercise program is more useful for people with permanent inner ear damage. It includes some exercise movements that can move crystals, and occasionally these particles will move toward the canal exit when Cawthorne exercises are performed. This means improvement in BPPV symptoms will take place eventually, but considerable time and many spells of vertigo can happen before any improvement occurs. The Cawthorne exercise program is therefore considered outdated and obsolete for the treatment of BPPV.

The Brandt–Daroff exercises are also described in Chapter 2, "The History of BPPV." The Brandt–Daroff exercises are very similar to the Semont maneuver, in that the patient moves from lying with one shoulder down to lying with the other shoulder down. However, in the Semont maneuver, the person's head faces the bed during the second half of the maneuver, while in the Brandt–Daroff exercises, the person ends up facing the ceiling. This small change means the particles are simply sloshed back and forth in the canal in the Brandt–Daroff exercises and only accidentally slip out of the canal. The outcome of the Brandt–Daroff exercises is similar to the Caw-thorne exercises: It takes too long to resolve symptoms and generates too much vertigo along the way.

Other Maneuvers for BPPV in the Horizontal Canal

In Chapter 9, "Unusual Forms of BPPV," we discussed the most effective maneuver for BPPV in the horizontal canal: the Gufoni maneuver. The most commonly used treatment for H-BPPV when administered by a provider is the Log Roll or Barbecue Roll maneuver and its many variations. In the Log Roll or Barbecue Roll maneuver, the patient starts by reclining on the side with the bad ear down and then rolls to the back, then to the other side, and finally to a face-down position on the bed. Usually this is done with a provider present, who helps the patient quickly rotate through the positions.

The Log Roll or Barbecue Roll can remove crystals from the horizontal canal, but it has several drawbacks. Recall from Chapter 9, "Unusual Forms of BPPV," that H-BPPV usually is triggered during maneuvers for the posterior canal such as the Epley maneuver and is caused by particles falling into the horizontal canal during subsequent attempts at the Dix–Hallpike maneuver. As discussed in Chapter 9, the simplest treatment is to immediately sit back up, preventing particles from falling deeply into the canal. Sitting up is the start of the Gufoni maneuver, and often this is all it takes to resolve H-BPPV. In contrast, the Log Roll or Barbecue Roll maneuver keeps the patient lying down, so the particles end up penetrating deeper into the horizontal canal. This is a serious limitation of the Log Roll or Barbecue Roll maneuver. It is also awkward to rotate the entire body in the Log Roll, instead of just rotating the head as is done in the Gufoni maneuver. For these reasons we no longer use the Log Roll or Barbecue Roll maneuver in my practice.

Some researchers have tried an alternative very simple method to remove crystals from the horizontal canal: holding the patient's head and shaking it briskly back and forth. This can help get particles out of the ampulla (see Chapter 9, "Unusual Forms of BPPV") but can also cause particles to enter the ampulla if they are not already in it, so it's better to use the Gufoni maneuver when first treating H-BPPV. At this point in the book, we've worked our way through how to do the Half Somersault as a home exercise and described maneuvers for a variety of BPPV problems. Most of the time, maneuvers allow you to completely resolve your vertigo. BPPV has one annoying characteristic, however: It returns. The next chapter provides tips to help reduce the number of BPPV recurrences.

11

Preventing Recurrences of BPPV

Sam writes:

❝I've had BPPV on and off over the past year (diagnosed by the Vestibular Clinic at Mass General), including three episodes of vertigo recurring a few days apart over the past two weeks. In this most recent 'series,' the spins stop after I do the Half Somersault maneuver a few times, but then the vertigo comes back after a few days (the same side, in bed at night, with relatively mild spins). My question is: Should I do the Half Somersault maneuver before I go to bed (or even multiple times per day) for some time after the vertigo is better to prevent recurrence?❞

Learning how to do maneuvers to remove particles is not enough to keep you permanently safe from a BPPV episode. You need to know how to keep the crystals in your ears in place where they belong so you don't experience repeated vertigo spells. Anyone who has ever had BPPV is eager to never have it again—no one wants to experience vertigo if they can prevent it from happening. The prevention of repeat BPPV spells is the subject of this chapter.

Performing the Half Somersault maneuver and removing particles that are in the incorrect place stops vertigo spells, but there is no "residual" effect to the "cure." It's possible to move your head in a way that will immediately reverse your success and put all those particles back in the wrong place just as soon as you finish. Luckily there are steps you can take to make that a lot less likely.

When you sit up at the end of a successful exercise, a mass of particles rolls out of the canal and into an open space or sac. At the side and bottom of this space lies the gravity sensor with a pile of still-attached particles on it. The clumps you have just removed and the particles on the sensor are all sticky and tend to cling to each other in general, but right at that moment (when you have just finished a maneuver) they are separated by fluid. If you put your head upside down, that loose clump is just the right size and shape to fall precisely back into the canals. To prevent this, you need to give the clump a chance to drift downward and stick back to its sibling particles on the sensor before you risk putting your head in certain positions.

Know When to Hold 'Em and Know When to Fold 'Em

Like a poker player, you need to know when to stop playing. Once the clumps are all out, doing one more maneuver can let those particles roll right back in. This is less of an issue with the Half Somersault than with other maneuvers primarily because the Dix–Hallpike position is much more likely to cause this and the Half Somersault does not include the Dix–Hallpike maneuver. If you do one too many Half Somersault maneuvers, any unintentionally dislodged otoconia particles will just fall right back out again at the end of the maneuver, so you'll probably lose nothing but your time.

Sometimes you feel completely restored at the end of a maneuver, with a sudden and dramatic absence of dizziness. If that happens, don't do another maneuver. You've probably gotten all the loose crystals out. If you're nauseated, though, it might be hard to tell if you are better and if the loose crystals are all out. If all the particles are out, you won't be able to make yourself spin by moving your head when you are upright. The easiest way to check this is to very quickly jerk your head up and down (like nodding quickly). Do you feel perfectly normal when you do that, or is there any kind of spinning or twisting feeling? If this jerky movement does not make your dizziness return, you should stop doing maneuvers at this point. If there is still a bit of dizziness, though, it is probably safe to do another maneuver.

Is the Vertigo Gone for Good?

If you have just experienced vertigo for the first time, once a treatment makes the spells stop, you may be able to go a very long time before another spell happens. A single occurrence is often just a case of bad luck. Many people can go years after a treatment without taking any special precautions. However, other people seem to risk moving the particles back in the canal every time they lie down. These people must be much more careful than other people. A third group of people fall in the middle: They have repeat spells but at least get a break for a few months or more in between spells.

Otoconia crystals are sticky and ideally should stick back down to the other crystals on the sensor once they have time to settle down, but in a lot of people this doesn't happen. The sticky coating on the crystals might be like the adhesive on an old Post-it note that just won't stick anymore. Some studies claim that old, broken crystals get reabsorbed by the body, but the many people with frequent recurrences prove that old crystals never go away.

People whose BPPV came on after a blow to the head, say in a car accident, are much more likely to get future attacks.[1] This is probably because a lot of particles get dislodged in the heads of people who are struck hard compared to the relatively few particles that are loose in people whose otoconia have jostled out of place naturally. If you've had more than one spell of BPPV already, then you are likely to have more. Repeated occurrences are an indicator that many of your particles are already loose and have trouble sticking back down.

Causes of Recurrence

The number one cause of frequent BPPV recurrences is having bad head-motion habits. Of course, you shouldn't blame yourself—these habits are only bad once you start getting BPPV. Before that, they were perfectly normal! The human head is very poorly designed to be placed upside down (see Chapter 3, "How Does Vertigo Happen?" p. 35). Animals have evolved to do best when they are strictly upright; for most animals that means even sleeping with their heads upright.

Humans, however, unlike most animals, like to sleep on their backs with their noses in the air, and do this almost every night. Many of us also do flips, somersault, roll down hills, practice yoga, get fillings at the dentist, and do sit-ups. All of these behaviors have the potential to set off BPPV. As discussed in Chapter 3, the human tendency to get BPPV is the result of an anatomic accident. If animals had been doing these movements for tens of millions of years, evolution might have worked out a new design to prevent us from getting particles in the wrong place. BPPV doesn't regularly stop humans from successfully mating or thriving, so it isn't that important in an evolutionary sense. For this reason, our ears are designed in a way that allows particles to mistakenly enter the canals whenever the head is horizontal or below the horizontal.

The worst thing to do if you are prone to BPPV is to place your head upside down. Yoga instructors may start getting BPPV, and their older clients may also notice some dizziness after vigorous sessions that include inverted positions such as downward dog. Flipping your head upside down to dry your hair is also a good way to trigger BPPV. Getting a shampoo at the salon can also be a problem if your head is tipped too far back into the bowl and then gets shaken around when your hair is shampooed. People that make a lot of high-acceleration/deceleration head movements playing sports are also more likely to shake particles loose. Mechanics that lie on their backs under cars to do repairs are another at-risk group. Doing flip turns in the pool or even turning the head side to side while swimming can trigger BPPV.

But even actions that you don't do regularly can trigger BPPV. If you crawl under your desk to retrieve a pen or look under a counter to fix a faucet, just having your head partly upside down and turned for that one event can start an episode of BPPV.

So what are the most common triggers? Moving or shaking the head while in certain positions can set off a series of attacks. Rolling over in bed is the most common way to set off a recurrence. The movement of fluid in the ear can jostle particles, and if the head is tipped back, gravity can pull them into a canal. A good way to cause a recurrence is to lie on your back with your head a little lower than your back, or with your chin tipped up a bit. If your head is turned slightly to one side when lying flat, a bout of BPPV is especially likely. Think about the position the dentist puts you in to drill or clean your teeth. A lot of people first experience vertigo in the dental chair, because not only is the position optimal for it, but the dentist also can apply drills and cleaning tools close to your ears that vibrate in a way that dislodges otoconia particles. Undergoing a surgery on some part of your head is also a risk, especially if vibrating drills are used. In any type of surgery, the head may be placed flat for anesthesia and then jiggled about. Some people awaken after surgery with BPPV.

Taking Precautions

After treating patients, I always advise them to prop up on at least two pillows when in bed and to avoid lying on the side with the bad ear for a week. This helps prevent recurrences for the week after the maneuver and ensures that the particles were successfully removed. However, after that week is up, recurrences can happen at any time. If a person is experiencing frequent bouts, sometimes simply learning to always sleep with the head propped on two pillows can be enough to prevent them.

Most people experience recurrences when in bed, so if you tend to wake up a bit when rolling over in the night, try to remember to lift your head off the pillow as you roll. Just raising your head a few inches is often high enough to prevent the particles from re-entering a canal. Always use one or two big pillows fluffed under your head if you lie on your back or side. If you are facing the ceiling, you probably have your head tipped too far back. You should face forward a bit and be looking at the top of the wall, not the ceiling.

Your head should never be moved beyond the horizontal plane either forward or backward (Figure 11.1). If you need to pick something up off of the floor, kneel down to get it so that you don't flip your head downward past the horizontal plane. Try not to do upside down positions in yoga or to lie flat in Pilates class. Yoga instructors who can't avoid these positions can do the Half Somersault at the end of a session to clear any particles that have moved out of place from the canals.

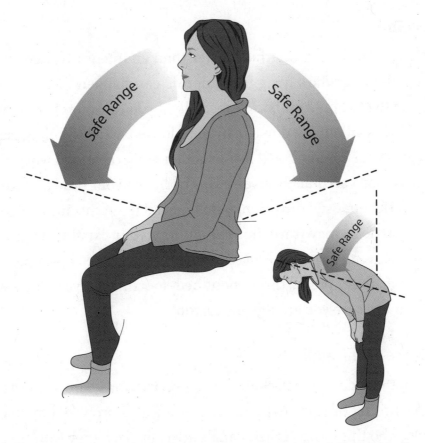

Figure 11.1   Safe head positions for BPPV. The head should be relatively upright as much as possible. Tipping forward to face the floor, or backward to face the ceiling, can cause particles to fall into the canals.

Tell the dentist you are prone to vertigo and ask the hygienist and the dentist to tip the exam chair up so your head remains above the horizontal. At the salon, tuck your chin down while your hair is shampooed so your head is not tilted too far back. If a surgery is planned, tell your anesthesiologist about your vertigo. If your head can be turned so that your bad ear is facing up, your risk of experiencing BPPV after surgery will be reduced.

Pillow Talk

Nothing ruins a sexy interlude faster than an intense vertigo spell, but for the one who's lying face up, this can happen distressingly often. Lying flat on your back, especially if you tip your chin up and to the side while lying down, can send loose particles rolling right back into your canals. You'll feel a sudden burst of vertigo when this happens. You can quickly reverse this by lifting your head and turning it in the opposite direction, but you need to do this immediately or the particles may travel far enough into your canal to require a full maneuver. A safer alternative is to keep your head propped up on a large, fluffy pillow throughout bed-sporting activities or, even better, make sure you are the one on top.

An Ounce of Prevention?

Why not just do the Half Somersault every day (as Sam suggests at the beginning of this chapter)? This is an idea proposed by many people, who think that if their canals are kept clean they won't experience a vertigo spell. Of course, if you lie down on your back and flip your head back while moving it around, it doesn't matter if you already did a maneuver that day: Particles can just fall right back in and the vertigo can come back that very second. If you keep getting BPPV, you should be careful what you do with your head all the time.

Doing maneuvers puts your head upside down and shakes it around, so even maneuvers can stir up the crystals. For this reason, it's probably best to leave well enough alone and not perform regular preventative maneuvers. On the other hand, particles probably build up in people gradually, too; a couple chunks here or there fall in while you are asleep until suddenly there is a large enough clump to trigger vertigo. Doing maneuvers to keep these from building up can, in theory, help prevent more violent recurrences.

What makes the most sense is to put off performing maneuvers until you feel at least a twinge of dizziness. If you roll over or tip your head back quickly and feel a second of swirling, this is a sign that some particles are starting to build up. Do a maneuver and afterward try a jerky nodding head movement as a test to see if the problem is improved. If you're not dizzy, then wait until you have another spell of dizziness before doing another maneuver. This won't stop particles from accidentally rolling back in, but it will keep them from building up.

In the next chapter, we will discuss common questions and review complications patients encountered in the course of BPPV treatment.

12

Troubleshooting

The preceding chapters have introduced you to BPPV and how it can be treated at home with the Half Somersault maneuver and other maneuvers. Over the years, my patients have asked questions about the Half Somersault maneuver, and other people have emailed me about the videos I have posted online. In this chapter, I answer the most common questions and concerns that people have when treating BPPV at home.

I don't know which side to treat. How can I tell?

Determining which ear is affected is covered in Chapter 7, "The Half Somersault Maneuver," so you may want to review the material on pp. 106–109. What follows is a short summary of that information: If the dizziness is worse when your right ear is down on the pillow, or when you roll from left to right in bed, the right ear is the likely cause. If the dizziness is worse when the left ear is down, or when you roll from right to left in bed, then the left ear is likely to be the problem. Some people have BPPV in both ears. If you aren't sure which ear it is or think it might be in both ears, try treating the worst side first by doing three to five maneuvers on that side. If the symptoms haven't gone away fully once you have completed the three to five maneuvers on the first side, then wait 15 minutes and do maneuvers for the opposite ear. Another choice is to do a maneuver for the right ear, then the left ear, alternating until symptoms are gone.

My spinning is worse the second or third repetition of the Half Somersault maneuver. Am I doing something wrong?

The amount of spinning you feel is determined by the number of particles that are moving as a clump in your canal. Larger clumps trigger more spinning. Often it takes more than one maneuver to dislodge the particles, which can get hung up in the canal. It's perfectly normal to experience a renewed, stronger burst of vertigo when a stuck clump suddenly comes loose. This often means that the particular maneuver you are doing is working and will be more successful.

I don't feel any spinning during the Half Somersault maneuver. Is it working?

The Half Somersault maneuver causes less intense spinning than other maneuvers because the particles are slowed down by a cushion of fluid for the first few seconds of the upside-down part of the maneuver. Particles can still be moved out even if you feel no dizziness, but you will likely have to repeat the maneuver more times to get completely clear if the first few times don't trigger a spinning sensation. Sometimes the particles adhere to the sides of the canal and have trouble starting their journey toward the exit. You can help mobilize the particles by tapping with your fingertip on the bone behind your ear, or putting something that vibrates against that area. Even a vibrating electric toothbrush handle pressed behind the ear can help get particles moving.

I get sick to my stomach while doing maneuvers. Is that normal?

Oddly enough, the center in the brain that controls vomiting is connected to the inner ears, which is why motion can make people seasick or carsick. BPPV creates a very strong feeling of movement, and if your BPPV is severe and you provoke the spinning several times in a row, you may experience nausea. If this happens, stop doing maneuvers until the nausea subsides, which usually takes 30 minutes. To prevent nausea from happening, you can try taking a non-prescription, over-the-counter (OTC) pill for motion sickness an hour before trying the Half Somersault maneuver. Meclizine, diphenhydramine, and dimenhydrinate are common OTC medications for nausea. Prescription medications for anxiety (tranquilizer benzodiazepines, such as Valium and Xanax) can also help.

I'm too scared to try the Half Somersault maneuver. Can a maneuver make my vertigo worse?

You have to be physically capable of making the head movements of the exercise to complete any maneuver safely. The Half Somersault maneuver is effective for BPPV and does not have any effect on other inner ear disorders; it can't make other ear diseases worse. The dizziness that occurs when crystals move can cause nausea and you can feel bad temporarily, but it does no harm to your inner ears or brain. The spinning you feel during the Half Somersault maneuver is simply a bad feeling that lasts for less than a minute. The amount of dizziness you feel while doing the Half Somersault maneuver is usually less than you would feel if a doctor or therapist performed the maneuvers on you discussed in Chapter 10, "Maneuvers Performed by a Provider." Nausea tends to last longer than the spinning feeling, but it usually resolves within half an hour. Taking a medicine for motion sickness can make this more tolerable (see the preceding question).

My nystagmus never stops. Is constant spinning a symptom of BPPV?

The Half Somersault and other maneuvers are only effective for BPPV, which causes very short but repeated spells of spinning lasting less than a minute. If you can see the environment spinning about you and this spinning is constant without stopping, it means you probably have a problem other than BPPV. For example, a person with a viral infection of the inner ear may see the room spin for several days in a row without stopping. Meniere's disease, a serious inner ear disorder, can cause spinning along with hearing loss and ringing in the ear that goes on for hours. If you have a strong headache with your dizziness, the problem may be migraine. See Chapter 4, "Non-BPPV Causes of Vertigo," for some common vertigo diseases that cannot be resolved with maneuvers. If your spinning does not stop, see a physician.

If my dizziness does not respond to maneuvers, what kind of provider should I see?

Dizziness can be evaluated by your primary care provider, but it is a complex problem and often referral to a specialist will be necessary. Physicians who specialize in the inner ear (otologists) and those who specialize in the brain (neurologists) are usually able to help. University-affiliated schools of medicine typically have experts in these areas on staff. Contact the closest medical school, if you are having trouble finding a provider to help you. There are also many physical therapists (PTs) and audiologists that provide help with maneuvers and treatment for balance problems resulting from inner ear disease. Look for a PT or audiologist specializing in vestibular rehabilitation.

I am terrified to drive because I have BPPV. Is it safe?

BPPV attacks usually only occur when making large vertical movements of the head. For example, they are most commonly triggered when you lie down in bed, arise from bed, or tip your head sharply up or down. Most people do not make these head movements while driving and so do not experience BPPV while in the car. BPPV can be triggered if the road is exceptionally bumpy, but the symptoms are usually only momentary in this case. Most people with BPPV continue driving, but if you are unable to turn your head to the side quickly or keep your vision stable, you should avoid driving. You should not drive if you see the environment spinning when you are upright, because this usually indicates another, more serious, inner ear problem that can impair driving.

The maneuver worked but didn't last. The vertigo came back a few days later. Why?

Maneuvers only remove particles from the canals. They can't stop the particles from going back into the canals later. Whether or not the particles re-enter the canals depends upon what you do with your head. Any time your head is tipped down so you are looking straight down at the floor, or backward far enough that you are looking straight up at the ceiling, you are in a position that allows particles access to the canals. Any time the top of your head is directed toward the floor, particles can enter the canals. People who have frequent recurrences should avoid all of these movements. The problem of recurrences and how to prevent them is covered in more detail in Chapter 11, "Preventing Recurrences of BPPV."

Do I have to be careful with head positions for the rest of my life or only the first few days after doing a maneuver?

After an episode of BPPV, it is a good idea to keep your head elevated on pillows when in bed and to avoid sleeping with the affected ear down for a few days to a week after doing maneuvers. This gives the loose particles time to drift away from the entrance to the canals and settle down on the sensor. However, if you have frequent recurrences, you may want to elevate your head when lying down for the rest of your life. An adjustable bed is a great help in this situation.

I teach yoga and can't give up my profession, but I keep getting BPPV. What can I do?

In general, people with recurrent BPPV should avoid doing upside-down head movements or exercises such as sit-ups. However, if your occupation demands that you perform these movements, you can utilize the Half Somersault maneuver to help prevent some recurrences. After doing a yoga session, perform the Half Somersault maneuver to remove any particles that might have become misplaced while exercising (see Chapter 11, "Preventing Recurrences of BPPV," p. 167, for more information on BPPV prevention).

I can't tolerate getting on my knees into the Half Somersault position. Is there an option for me?

As discussed in Chapter 8, "Variations of the Half Somersault Maneuver," the Half Somersault maneuver can be done while you are seated, lying on your stomach, or even while you are standing. If none of these positions can be tolerated, you may want to try using the Semont maneuver (see Chapter 10, "Maneuvers Performed by a Provider," p. 151).

When I moved into the upright position at the completion of the Half Somersault maneuver, I suddenly experienced very severe vertigo for several seconds. What happened?

When your head is moved to the upright position, particles should be flushed forward and toward the exit of the canal. Sometimes you can feel these particles leaving in the form of vertigo. This bout of vertigo usually lasts for just a second or two. However, if the particles were very deep in the canal and did not make it far enough around the curve during the maneuver, they can fall all the way back down into the bottom of the canal (Figure 12.1). When this happens, it causes vertigo that tends to last longer—as long as 20 or 30 seconds. These two types of vertigo may be difficult to tell apart. The simple

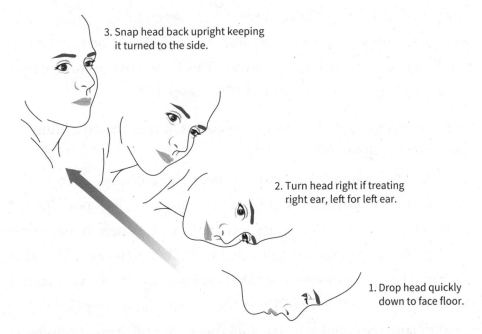

3. Snap head back upright keeping it turned to the side.

2. Turn head right if treating right ear, left for left ear.

1. Drop head quickly down to face floor.

Figure 12.1 Treatment for particles falling back in to the canal. (1 and 2) Tip the head downward to face the floor and turn your head toward the shoulder on the same side as the affected ear. (3) Wait 30 seconds, and then snap your head upright again, keeping it turned.

solution when you feel any sort of vertigo at the conclusion of the maneuver is to immediately tuck your chin to your chest so you are facing the floor. Turn your head so you are looking at the elbow on the same side that you were just treating. Wait at least 30 seconds and then snap your head upright again. After you have done this, move your head up and down to see if the dizziness is still present. If it is, do the maneuver again.

After I completed various BPPV maneuvers, the spinning has changed and is even worse. What is the matter?

All maneuvers carry a risk of moving particles throughout the ear. The Half Somersault maneuver is designed to reduce the risk of moving particles into the horizontal semicircular canal. The indication that your particles have entered another canal is a sudden dramatic worsening of vertigo that does not improve when using the Half Somersault or Epley maneuvers. This is covered in more detail in Chapter 9, "Unusual Forms of BPPV," on p. 127.

My dizziness changed after doing maneuvers. It was off and on but now it is continuous. What can I do?

You may have particles stuck in or near the ampulla, deep in the canal. If a lot of particles slip inside the ampulla, it is possible for them to form a clump that is larger than the exit. When they attempt to leave, they form a sort of ball-valve and lodge in the exit. This also can happen in places where the canal narrows, about halfway around the canal. When you have BPPV in the ampulla (ampullary BPPV) or canalith jam, the canal acts like it has been shut off. This condition is discussed in more detail and the maneuvers used to treat it are given in Chapter 9, "Unusual Forms of BPPV," p. 127.

Bibliography

Chapter 1

1. Foster CA, Ponnapan A, Zaccaro K, Strong D. A comparison of two home exercises for benign positional vertigo: Half somersault versus Epley maneuver. *Audiol Neurotol Extra* 2014; 2:16–23.

Chapter 2

1. von Brevern M, Radtke A, Lezius F, et al. Epidemiology of benign paroxysmal positional vertigo: A population based study. *J Neurol Neurosurg Psychiatry* 2007; 78:710–15.
2. Schuknecht HF. Positional vertigo: Clinical and experimental observations. *Trans Am Acad Ophthalmol Otolaryngol* 1962; 66:319–32.
3. Lowenstein O, Thornhill RA. *The labyrinth of myxine: Anatomy, ultrastructure and electrophysiology.* Proceedings of the Royal Society of London Series B Biological Sciences 1970; 176:21–42.
4. Mallory J, Adams D. *The Oxford introduction to Proto-Indo-European and the Proto-Indo-European world.* Oxford: Oxford University Press; 2006.
5. Bárány R. Diagnose von Krankheitsercheingungen im Bereiche de Otolithenapparates [Diagnosis of symptoms in the areas of Otolithenapparates]. *Acta Oto-Laryngol* 1921; 2:434–37.
6. Baloh RW. Robert Bárány and the controversy surrounding his discovery of the caloric reaction. *Neurology* 2002; 58:1094–99.
7. Dix MR, Hallpike CS. *The pathology symptomatology and diagnosis of certain common disorders of the vestibular system. Proc R Soc Med* 1952; 45:341–54.

8. Lanska DJ, Remler B. Benign paroxysmal positioning vertigo: Classic descriptions, origins of the provocative positioning technique, and conceptual developments. *Neurology* 1997; 48:1167–77.

9. Cooksey FS. *Rehabilitation in vestibular injuries. Proc R Soc Med* 1946; 39:273–78.

10. Dix, 7.

11. Lanska, 9.

12. Dix, 7.

13. Schuknecht HF. John R. Lindsay: Clinician, teacher, otopathologist. *Ann Otol Rhinol Laryngol Suppl* 1983; 102:12–16.

14. Hemenway WG, Lindsay JR. Postural vertigo due to unilateral sudden partial loss of vestibular function. *Ann Otol Rhinol Laryngol* 1956; 65:692–706.

15. Schuknecht, 2.

16. Schuknecht HF. Cupulolithiasis. *Arch Otolaryngol* 1969; 90:765–78.

17. Gacek RR. Transection of the posterior ampullary nerve for the relief of benign paroxysmal positional vertigo. *Ann Otol Rhinol Laryngol* 1974; 83:596–605.

18. Gacek RR, Gacek MR. Singular neurectomy in the management of paroxysmal positional vertigo. *Otolaryngol Clin North Am* 1994; 27:363–79.

19. Hall SF, Ruby RR, McClure JA. The mechanics of benign paroxysmal vertigo. *J Otolaryngol* 1979; 8:151–58.

20. Parnes LS, McClure JA. Free-floating endolymph particles: A new operative finding during posterior semicircular canal occlusion. *Laryngoscope* 1992; 102:988–92.

21. Brandt T, Daroff RB. Physical therapy for benign paroxysmal positional vertigo. *Arch Otolaryngol* 1980; 106:484–85.

22. Rojas-Burke J. Cursing the cure: Doctor and invention outlast jeers and threats. *The Oregonian* December 31, 2006.

23. Baloh RW. *Vertigo: Five physician scientists and the quest for a cure.* New York: Oxford University Press; 2017.

24. Epley JM. The canalith repositioning procedure: For treatment of benign paroxysmal positional vertigo. *Otolaryngol Head Neck Surg* 1992; 107:399–404.

25. Semont A, Freyss G, Vitte E. Curing the BPPV with a liberatory maneuver. *Adv Otorhinolaryngol* 1988; 42:290–93.

26. Ibid.

27. Parnes LS, McClure JA. Posterior semicircular canal occlusion for intractable benign paroxysmal positional vertigo. *Ann Otol Rhinol Laryngol* 1990; 99:330–34.

Chapter 3

1. Hudspeth AJ. Integrating the active process of hair cells with cochlear function. *Nat Rev Neurosci* 2014; 15:600–614.

2. Purves D, Augustine GJ, Fitzpatrick D, et al., eds. The otolith organs: The untricle and sacculus. *Neuroscience* 2e. Sunderland, MA: Sinauer; 2001.

3. Yakushin S, Dai M, Suzuki J, Raphan T, Cohen B. Semicircular canal contributions to the three-dimensional vestibuloocular reflex: A model-based approach. *J Neurophysiol* 1995; 74:2722–2738.

4. Baloh RW, Honrubia V. The Central Vestibular System. In *Clinical neurophysiology of the vestibular system*. New York, Oxford University Press; 1990.

5. Rajguru SM, Ifediba MA, Rabbitt RD. Three-dimensional biome-chanical model of benign paroxysmal positional vertigo. *Ann Biomed Eng* 2004; 32:831–46.

Chapter 4

1. Foster C. Unilateral sudden loss of vestibular function and vestibular neuritis. In: Dispenza F, De Stefano A, eds. *Vertigo: Diagnosis and management.* London: Jaypee Brothers Medical; 2013:115–27.

2. Johnson F, Semaan MT, Megerian CA. Temporal bone fracture: Evaluation and management in the modern era. *Otolaryngol Clin North Am* 2008; 41:597–618.

3. Kim HA, Lee H. Recent advances in understanding audiovestibular loss of a vascular cause. *J Stroke* 2017; 19:61–66.

4. Van Hecke R, Van Rompaey V, Wuyts FL, Leyssens L, Maes L. Systemic aminoglycosides-induced vestibulotoxicity in humans. *Ear Hear* 2017;38(6):653–662.

5. Nakashima T, Pyykkö I, Arroll MA, et al. Meniere's disease. *Nat Rev Dis Primers* 2016; 2:16028.

6. Foster CA, Breeze RE. The Meniere attack: An ischemia/reperfusion disorder of inner ear sensory tissues. *Med Hypotheses* 2013; 81:1108–1115.

7. Zalewski CK, Chien WW, King KA, et al. Vestibular dysfunction in patients with enlarged vestibular aqueduct. *Otolaryngol Head Neck Surg* 2015; 153:257–62.

8. Matsuoka AJ, Harris JP. Autoimmune inner ear disease: A retrospective review of forty-seven patients. *Audiol Neurootol* 2013; 18:228–39.

9. von Brevern M, Lempert T. Vestibular migraine. *Handb Clin Neurol* 2016; 137:301–16.

10. Charles A, Hansen JM. Migraine aura: New ideas about cause, classification, and clinical significance. *Curr Opin Neurol* 2015; 28:255–60.

11. Foster CA, Pollard CK. Comparison of caloric reactivity between migraineurs and non-migraineurs. *J Laryngol Otol* 2015; 129:960–63.

12. Tsai MS, Lee LA, Tsai YT, et al. Sleep apnea and risk of vertigo: A nationwide population-based cohort study. *Laryngoscope* 2018 Mar;128(3):763–68.

13. Ishiyama G, Ishiyama A, Baloh RW. Drop attacks and vertigo secondary to a non-meniere otologic cause. *Arch Neurol* 2003; 60:71–75.

Chapter 5

1. Fetter M, Haslwanter T, Bork M, Dichgans J. New insights into positional alcohol nystagmus using three-dimensional eye-movement analysis. *Ann Neurol* 1999; 45:216–23.

2. Imai T, Matsuda K, Takeda N, et al. Light cupula: The pathophysiological basis of persistent geotropic positional nystagmus. *BMJ Open* 2015; 5(1):e006607.

3. Horii A, Saika T, Uno A, et al. Factors relating to the vertigo control and hearing changes following intratympanic gentamicin for intractable Meniere's disease. *Otol Neurotol* 2006; 27:896–900.

4. Wu D, Thijs RD. Anticonvulsant-induced downbeat nystagmus in epilepsy. *Epilepsy Behav Case Rep* 2015; 4:74–5.

5. Halmagyi GM, Lessell I, Curthoys IS, Lessell S, Hoyt WF. Lithium-induced downbeat nystagmus. *Am J Ophthalmol* 1989; 107:664–70.

6. Nerrant E, Tilikete C. Ocular motor manifestations of multiple sclerosis. *J Neuroophthalmol* 2017; 37:332–40.

7. Doijiri R, Uno H, Miyashita K, Ihara M, Nagatsuka K. How Commonly is stroke found in patients with isolated vertigo or dizziness attack? *J Stroke Cerebrovasc Dis* 2016; 25:2549–2552.

8. Wessel K, Moschner C, Wandinger KP, Kompf D, Heide W. Oculomotor testing in the differential diagnosis of degenerative ataxic disorders. *Arch Neurol* 1998; 55:949–56.

9. Cho BH, Kim SH, Kim SS, Choi YJ, Lee SH. Central positional nystagmus associated with cerebellar tumors: Clinical and topographical analysis. *J Neurol Sci* 2017; 373:147–51.

10. Brandt T, Dieterich M. The dizzy patient: Don't forget disorders of the central vestibular system. *Nat Rev Neurol* 2017; 13:352–62.

Chapter 6

1. de Kleijn A, Magnus R. Ueber die funktion der otolithen [About the function of otoliths]. *Pflugers Arch Gesamte Physiol Menschen Tiere* 1921; 186:6–81.

2. Babac S, Djeric D, Petrovic–Lazic M, Arsovic N, Mikic A. Why do treatment failure and recurrences of benign paroxysmal positional vertigo occur? *Otol Neurotol* 2014; 35:1105–110.

3. Ibid.

Chapter 7

1. Foster CA, Ponnapan A, Zaccaro K, Strong D. A comparison of two home exercises for benign positional vertigo: Half somersault versus Epley maneuver. *Audiol Neurotol Extra* 2014; 2:16–23.

2. Ibid.

Chapter 9

1. Foster C, Zaccaro K, Strong D. Canal conversion and re-entry: A risk of Dix–Hallpike during canalith repositioning procedures. *Otol Neurotol* 2012; 33:199–203.

2. Korres S, Balatsouras DG, Kaberos A, Economou C, Kandiloros D, Ferekidis E. Occurrence of semicircular canal involvement in benign paroxysmal positional vertigo. *Otol Neurotol* 2002; 23:926–32.

3. Foster, 1.

4. Yacovino D, Hain T, Gualtieri F. New therapeutic maneuver for anterior canal benign paroxysmal positional vertigo. *J Neurol* 2009; 256:1851–55.

5. Ibid.

6. Lee S-U, Kim H-J, Kim J-S. Pseudo-spontaneous and head-shaking nystagmus in horizontal canal benign paroxysmal positional vertigo. *Otol Neurotol* 2014; 35:495–500.

7. Gufoni M, M. L. Tratiamento con manovra di reposizionamento per la canalolitiasi orrizontale. *Acta Otorhinolaringol Ital* 1998; 18: 363–367.

8. Yakovino, 4.

Chapter 10

1. Foster C, Zaccaro K, Strong D. Canal conversion and re-entry: A risk of Dix–Hallpike during canalith repositioning procedures. *Otol Neurotol* 2012; 33:199–203.

2. Epley JM. The canalith repositioning procedure: for treatment of benign paroxysmal positional vertigo. *Otolaryngology–Head and Neck Surgery* 1992; 107:399–404.

Chapter 11

1. Motin M, Keren O, Groswasser Z, Gordon CR. Benign paroxysmal positional vertigo as the cause of dizziness in patients after severe traumatic brain injury: Diagnosis and treatment. *Brain Inj* 2005; 19:693–97.

Index

Note: Page numbers followed by *f* or *t* indicate a figure or table.